THE COMPLETE GUIDE TO

BEATING
SUGAR
ADDICTION!

JT: TTo Laurie, my wife, my best friend, and the love of my life, and to my son Dave, daughters Amy, Shannon, Brittany, and Kelly, and grandkids Payton and Bryce, who seem to have been born knowing what I'm just learning.

CF: To my nephews Jake and Alex. I am blessed to have you in my life!

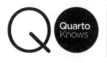

Quarto is the authority on a wide range of topics.

Quarto educates, entertains and enriches the lives of our readers—enthusiasts and lovers of hands-on living.

www.quartoknows.com

First published in the USA in 2015 by
Fair Winds Press, an imprint of
Quarto Publishing Group USA Inc.
100 Cummings Center
Suite 406-L
Beverly, MA 01915-6101
QuartoKnows.com
Visit our blogs at QuartoKnows.com

19 18 17 16   2 3 4 5

ISBN: 978-1-59233-678-4

Library of Congress Cataloging-in-Publication Data available

Cover design by Studioink.co.uk
Book design by Studioink.co.uk
Printed and bound in USA

The information in this book is for educational purposes only. It is not intended to replace the advice of a physician or medical practitioner. Please see your healthcare provider before beginning any new health program.

THE COMPLETE GUIDE TO
BEATING SUGAR ADDICTION!

The Cutting-Edge Program That Cures Your Type
of Sugar Addiction and Puts You Back on the
Road to Weight Control and Good Health

JACOB TEITELBAUM, M.D.
CHRYSTLE FIEDLER AND
DIERDRE RAWLINGS, PH.D., N.D.

FAIR WINDS

CONTENTS

INTRODUCTION: AN OVERVIEW OF SUGAR ADDICTION

Are you a sugar addict? If the answer is yes, you are not alone.

American adults consume about 15 percent of our calories from sugars that are added to foods during processing—or 140 to 150 pounds of sugar per person each year! A mind blowing 37 percent of added sugars are consumed in sugar-sweetened beverages, while another 18 percent of our calories come from white flour (which acts a lot like sugar in our bodies)! It's not surprising that we have become a nation of sugar addicts. Like many other addictive substances, sugar may leave you feeling a bit better for a few hours, but then it wreaks havoc on your body and can cause long-term health problems.

The good news? There is a solution that works. In this book, we will teach you about the four main types of sugar addicts. In each type, there are different forces driving the addiction, and in all four types, the excess sugar leaves people feeling much worse overall. By treating the underlying causes that are active in your type of addiction, you will find that not only do your sugar cravings go away, but you also feel dramatically better overall.

Here's more good news. Once you have broken your sugar addiction, your body will usually be able to handle sugar in moderation. This means saving sugar for dessert or snacks where it belongs and going for quality, not quantity. Dark chocolate is especially okay.

We will also discuss how to "have your cake and eat it too"—how to use natural sugar substitutes to get the pleasure without paying the cost. It is not our goal to eliminate things you love. Our goal instead is to teach you how to get the most pleasure you can, in a way that is healthy for your body and leaves you feeling better. In medicine, we have a simple rule: Never take away something pleasurable from a person's diet without substituting something equally pleasurable. Otherwise, it just doesn't work!

WHY IS SUGAR ADDICTIVE?

For thousands of years, humans ate sugar found naturally in their food. Sugar was not a problem; it was a treat. But now more than one-third of the calories we consume come from sugar and white flour added during food processing. Our bodies simply were not designed to handle this massive load.

Many of you have already noticed that although sugar gives you an initial high, you crash several hours later, and this leaves you wanting more sugar. In fact, sugar acts as an energy loan shark, taking away more energy than it gives. Eventually, your "credit line" runs out and you find yourself exhausted, anxious, and moody.

THE LONG-TERM CONSEQUENCES OF SUGAR ADDICTION

In addition to the immediate fatigue and emotional problems, the research shows that sugar also causes many long-term health problems. For example, according to a study published in the medical journal *Diabetologia* (2012), drinking just one 12-ounce (355 ml) sugar-sweetened soft drink a day can increase the risk of type 2 diabetes by 22 percent. While a study published in the medical journal *JAMA Internal Medicine* (2014) showed that just one can of soda a day ups heart attack risk by 30 percent. That's pretty scary stuff.

DANGEROUS SUGAR: HIGH FRUCTOSE CORN SYRUP

While all excess sugar is detrimental to your health, high fructose corn syrup, a mixture of fructose and glucose, often found in beverages, is the worst for you. In the U.S., the consumption of high-fructose corn syrup has risen 250 percent in the past fifteen years—and our rate of diabetes has increased approximately 45 percent during the same time period.

High fructose corn syrup is made by food refiners who turn cornstarch into sugary syrups that are then added to sodas, candy, cereal, bread, dairy products, and processed foods. Although the sugar industry sometimes tries to confuse the public by claiming that corn syrup is not sugar, it is a form of sugar as far as your body is concerned—and more toxic than cane sugar.

A study in the journal *Cancer Research* (2010) showed that pancreatic tumor cells actually use fructose, to divide and proliferate. This may help explain other studies that have linked fructose intake with pancreatic cancer.

HOW SUGAR CAUSES INFLAMMATION AND CHRONIC DISEASE

Too much sugar, white flour, and other refined carbohydrates in our diet—about 20 percent of our total calories—increase inflammation in the body. Inflammation can be acute, from an infection or after a cut or other injury, or chronic and can cause heart disease, stroke, and cancer.

Your immune system's job is to protect you from outside invaders. Antibodies are a type of protein that detects invaders and sees them as "other" so that immune cells, like white blood cells and natural killer cells, can recognize and kill them. When this happens, inflammation results, which can be a good thing, a protective response by the body that helps you heal.

However, if inflammation lasts too long and becomes chronic, it can actually damage the tissues of your body. In your arteries, for example, your immune system responds to cholesterol as a foreign invader. White blood cells inflame the arterial lining and form plaque. When it becomes chronic, this inflammation is the key factor behind the plaque buildup that causes heart disease and stroke —the #1 and #3 killers of Americans.

CHRONIC MEDICAL PROBLEMS ASSOCIATED WITH SUGAR IN OUR DIET:

- Chronic fatigue syndrome and fibromyalgia

- Pain of many kinds

- Decreased immune function

- Chronic sinusitis

- Irritable bowel syndrome and spastic colon

- Autoimmune disease

- Cancer

- Metabolic syndrome with high cholesterol and hypertension

- Heart disease

- Hormonal problems

- Schizophrenia

- Candida and yeast infections

- ADHD

This is the short list. The actual list could go on for pages! Sugar is also a mood-altering substance, causing stress, anxiety, and depression, which is no surprise to anyone with a sweet tooth. For all these reasons, it's likely that if sugar growers tried to win FDA approval today, they'd have a tough time getting permission to sell their product.

But the fact is, sugar is everywhere in our diet, and it is dumped into what we eat and drink during food processing. With one-third of our calories coming from sugar and white flour, and the stress of modern life increasing, we are seeing the makings of the "perfect storm" of medical problems. Eating sugar causes blood sugar to surge, insulin to spike, and fat to get deposited throughout your body. Obesity, often accompanied by diabetes and heart disease, is just one more consequence of our high-sugar diet.

THE VALUE OF SUGAR DETOX

I know the value of ridding the body of excess sugar. For more than thirty years, I have incorporated sugar detox into treatments for countless patients suffering from chronic health problems. I have also seen thousands of people whose chronic fatigue syndrome and fibromyalgia were aggravated by a sweet tooth.

I also understand the problem firsthand. A former sugar addict myself, I came down with chronic fatigue syndrome in 1975. Eliminating my sugar addiction was an important part of my recovery.

Sugar addiction is the canary in the coal mine. It usually points to a larger problem that is also dragging you down. We don't have anything against sugar. We simply don't want you feeling poorly and getting sick because of it. In fact, we want you to feel great! And most of you will when you treat the problems accompanying your sugar addiction. Ready to get off the "sugar roller coaster?" We're happy to guide the way.

The basics of sugar detox are, of course, diet related (stop eating sugar), and diet alteration is the standard method used to overcome sugar addiction. But an even deeper level of treatment is necessary to produce wellness. If you have tried the "cold turkey" approach to sugar addiction without nutritional strategies, treatment guidelines, and support, you probably found success elusive. That's because getting rid of the sugar is but one step in an overall comprehensive approach that must address the mind, body, and spirit.

The most successful way to treat sugar addition includes a process called medical triage. This means addressing the relative severity of each problem and then organizing treatment in order of priority. The problem with many medical self-help books is that they pick off a little corner of the problem and miss the big picture, so often you get frustrated and stop your program without getting well. My goal in writing is to give you an organized approach, so you can effectively kick sugar addiction—along with the hidden problems driving your addiction.

This book gives you a step-by-step approach for each type of sugar addiction that encourages you to change from a sugar-laden to a low-sugar diet without sacrificing the pleasures of food and eating. Although I will offer suggestions, I believe in personalized medicine; therefore, this book takes a flexible, real-life approach to becoming sugar healthy. Although we will offer guidelines for healthy eating, sugar substitution, and treatments to aid withdrawal and heal the body, we encourage you most of all to trust your intuition and listen to your body as you recover and see what makes you feel the best.

THE FOUR TYPES OF SUGAR ADDICTION

To beat sugar addiction, first you'll need to figure out which type of sugar addict you are. Think of it like a road trip. The initial step is to decide the best way to get to where you want to be: free of sugar addiction and feeling great. Consider this book as your road map to wellness. We include directions for your inner journey, a journey that will heal not only your body but also your mind and spirit. A journey that will change your life!

Different kinds of sugar addiction have different underlying causes and require different treatments. Here are the four key types of sugar addiction:

Type 1: The Energy Loan Shark

Chronically exhausted and hooked on quick hits of caffeine and sugar

When daily fatigue causes sugar (and caffeine) cravings, sometimes all you need is to improve nutrition, sleep, and exercise. When your energy increases, you won't need sugar and as much caffeine for an energy boost. New research shows that coffee can be beneficial when used in moderation, and we'll show you how. You'll find out how to turbocharge your energy in an easy and healthy way starting in chapter 1.

Type 2: Feed Me Now or I'll Kill You

When life's stress has exhausted your adrenal glands

For those of you who get irritable when you're hungry and crash under stress, it is important to treat your adrenal exhaustion. You'll learn how to nourish your adrenals and beat this type of sugar addiction, for good, beginning in chapter 2.

Type 3: The Happy Ho-Ho Hunter

Sugar cravings caused by yeast/candida overgrowth

For those of you with chronic nasal congestion, sinusitis, spastic colon, or irritable bowel syndrome, treating yeast overgrowth is critical. Learn all about probiotics, healing sugar addiction, and begin to take steps to wellness in chapter 3.

Type 4: Depressed and Craving Carbs

Sugar cravings caused by your period, menopause, or andropause

For women who feel worse around their menstrual cycle, or whose problems increased when they entered perimenopause in their forties, and during menopause, estrogen and progesterone deficiency may be driving your sugar craving. In a woman's earlier years, this is likely to reflect as premenstrual syndrome (PMS, with associated progesterone deficiency), with severe irritability around your periods. In your mid-forties, as estrogen deficiency begins, estrogen or progesterone deficiency often produces increased sugar cravings, fatigue, moodiness, and insomnia around your periods, as well as decreased vaginal lubrication.

For men, testosterone deficiency associated with andropause can also cause sugar craving, along with other severe problems. Depression, decreased libido, decreased erectile function, high blood pressure, weight gain, diabetes, or high cholesterol can suggest testosterone deficiency. Interestingly, supplementing with bio-identical natural testosterone (by prescription) has been shown to help all of these problems.

Standard blood testing for hormonal deficiencies will not reveal the problems until they are very severe, sometimes leaving people deficient for decades. Find out why eliminating sugar addiction and other problems caused by low estrogen, progesterone, or testosterone is essential, starting in chapter 4.

HOW TO USE THIS BOOK

To make it easy, we have structured this book as a workbook, so that when you're done reading it, you will have a treatment protocol tailored to your specific problems.

Part I consists of four chapters that will help you learn about the four types of sugar addiction. Each chapter is devoted to a specific type. To find out which type of sugar addict you are, the first step is to take the quiz at the beginning of each chapter. Your score will tell you which type of sugar addiction you have. You may have more than one. The next step is to go to Part II to learn about the treatment protocols for each type.

Part II features five chapters that focus on healing strategies for all sugar addicts beginning with bonus educational materials to help you really understand the problem of sugar addiction. After that, move on to the most important part—the treatments for each of the four types of sugar addiction. As you go through the chapters, you will create a treatment protocol tailored to your individual type of sugar addiction by checking off the wellness prescription treatments you need in addition to items in appendix A. When you get to the end of the book, you'll have a treatment protocol tailored to your own individual addiction type! Think of it as DIY health, with the goal of making you sugar-free!

Part III offers concise guidance for treating specific problems associated with sugar addiction, including chronic fatigue syndrome, fibromyalgia, spastic colon, sinusitis, diabetes, and more.

Ready to get a life you love? Read on to find out how.

Love and blessings,

Jacob Teitelbaum, MD

PART 1

THE PROBLEM

Part 1 is composed of four chapters that describe the four different types of sugar addicts. To find out which type you are, just take the brief quiz at the beginning of each chapter. If your score qualifies you for that type, you'll need to follow the wellness prescription found in part II for that sugar addiction type. If your score doesn't qualify you as a particular type of sugar addict, move on to the next chapter. If you have more than one type, you'll follow the wellness prescriptions for both types in part II. Ready to kick the sugar habit, feel great, and get the life you love? Good! Let's get started!

1

TYPE 1 SUGAR ADDICTION: THE ENERGY LOAN SHARK

Chronically exhausted and hooked on quick hits of caffeine and sugar

Type 1 sugar addicts are addicted to energy drinks, coffee, and/or soft drinks containing caffeine. Energy drinks have grown in popularity since Red Bull was introduced in 1997. Today there are more than 500 energy drinks on the market, which together account for more than $5.7 billion in sales. The basic ingredients in most energy drinks are sugar and caffeine (although some brands add herbal extracts, amino acids such as taurine, and vitamins). When this mixture of empty calories hits your system and your blood sugar rises, you get an immediate energy boost. Unfortunately, one to three hours later you feel even more fatigued than before. You also crave more sugar. What do you do? Reach for another energy drink. Fatigue drives sugar cravings, and sugar consumption drives fatigue. Getting energy from "energy drinks" (including coffee and sodas) is like borrowing money from a loan shark—it costs you way more in the end.

TAKE THIS QUIZ

Your total score will tell you whether you fit the type 1 profile. Do you?

_____	Do you feel tired much of the time? (20 points)
_____	Do you need coffee to get jumpstarted in the morning? (10 points)
✗	Do you experience a mid-afternoon slump? (10 points)
_____	Do you have occasional insomnia? (20 points)
✗	Do you have indigestion? (15 points)
✗	Do you feel achy? (15 points)
_____	Do you have frequent headaches? (15 points)
_____	Are you gaining weight? Or having trouble losing weight? (Score 1 point for every two pounds gained over the past three years.)
_____	What is the average number of ounces of caffeinated coffee or soda you drink daily? (Score 2 points for each ounce.)
_____	What is the average number of ounces of "energy drinks" containing sugar or caffeine that you drink daily? (Score 6 points for each ounce.)
_____	Do you repeatedly crave sweets or caffeine to give you the energy to get through the day? (25 points)
_____	Are you working more than forty hours a week? (Score 2 points for each hour over forty.)
_____	Your total score

SCORE	
0–40:	No problem. Skip to the quiz at the beginning of the next chapter.
41–70:	The tips in this chapter will help you restore your energy production.
Over 70:	You are a sugar and caffeine junkie. Read on to learn how to restore your energy production naturally, so you can cut back on sugar and still feel great.

WHAT DOES A TYPICAL TYPE 1 SUGAR ADDICT LOOK LIKE?

If you're a type 1 sugar addict, it's likely you are a type A personality, which means you strive for perfection. Nothing less than the best you can do is acceptable. Whether you are a college student pulling all-nighters, a Young Turk climbing the corporate ladder, or a woman working on breaking the glass ceiling, your attention is focused with laser-like precision on success.

Chances are you work (or want to work) in a highly competitive field such as law, medicine, high finance, or high tech. But you can be a type 1 sugar addict regardless of your work situation (yes, stay-at-home moms count). The common denominator of all type 1 sugar addicts is that there never seems to be enough hours in the day to get everything done. Downtime is not on your to-do list, and fatigue is ever present.

If you try to exercise, you are plagued with aches and pains because your muscles just don't have the energy they need to function properly. If you skip a workout, muscles tighten, causing pain, and when this becomes chronic, it is called fibromyalgia.

Low energy can also cause muscle tightness in the neck and shoulders, a factor in tension headaches and/or migraines. Caffeine withdrawal (even if it's temporary) and even an allergy to sugar can also trigger migraines.

It's not unusual for a type 1 sugar addict to have hypothyroidism. When your thyroid gland (located in your neck), the master of metabolism, isn't working the way it should, fatigue results. This further perpetuates a dependence on energy drinks to boost energy artificially.

MORE HEALTH PROBLEMS COMMON TO TYPE 1 SUGAR ADDICTS

Often, the type 1 sugar addict has a weakened immune system. Repeatedly pumping sugar into your body with energy drinks puts you at a deficit for certain essential nutrients, such as zinc, which you need for proper immune function. When you don't get the nutrients you need, your body's defense system becomes impaired. In fact, the sugar in one can of soda can immediately decrease your immune function by one-third for three to four hours!

Do you seem to catch every illness that's going around, and then it takes forever for the infection to go away? If so, your immune system may be sluggish. You may get viral infections, such as a cold or flu, or have chronic sore throats. In more severe cases, immune dysfunction can be associated with infections that should be short term but become chronic, such as Epstein-Barr syndrome.

Chronic use of energy drinks to boost energy artificially wreaks havoc on the body and can lead to all sorts of problems, including sugar addiction, fatigue, insulin resistance, weight gain, chronic fatigue syndrome (CFS), and fibromyalgia (FMS). Over the past ten years, research has shown that the incidence of chronic fatigue syndrome and fibromyalgia has increased by 400 to 1,000 percent, with more than 12 million Americans (three-quarters of them female) being affected. More than 25 million Americans suffer from chronic *disabling* fatigue, and most people feel they simply don't have enough energy. We will discuss how to recover from these debilitating illnesses in part III.

The Effects Energy Drinks Can Have on Your Heart

Research done in 2007 at the Henry Ford Hospital in Detroit, Michigan, showed that energy drinks with caffeine and taurine can increase heart rate and blood pressure levels, a potential problem for people who have heart disease or hypertension. Other side effects of caffeine include nervousness, irritability, insomnia, and chronic headaches. You'll find more information about the harmful effects of sugar addiction in chapter 5: Healing Practices for All Sugar Addicts.

THE TYPE 1 SUGAR ADDICT'S DIET

Type 1 sugar addicts often eat on the run, usually fast foods that contain sugar, fat, and salt, because you don't have enough time to sit down for a real meal. Because of this, you lack vitamins and minerals that are essential for energy production, such as B vitamins (B_1, B_2, B_3, B_5, B_6, and B_{12}), magnesium, and zinc, which are critical to immune function—which is one reason why you get sick so often.

White flour and white rice (which have essentially been stripped of nutrients and are easily converted into sugar in the body) supply another major part of your diet. In fact, more than one-third of the calories in the average American's diet come from sugar and white flour—a whopping 35 percent of what you eat provides essentially no vitamins or minerals. Eating these empty calories is like having a third of your paycheck bounce!

A nutrient-poor diet translates into an energy deficit. You won't have the building blocks you need for vital bodily functions, including burning calories to generate energy, repairing tissue, making "happiness molecules" such as serotonin, and keeping your brain working optimally. The type 1 sugar addict's lose-lose solution is to reach for a quick energy fix in the form of an energy drink packed with sugar and caffeine.

Eventually, eating the wrong foods and eating on the run causes acid reflux and indigestion, a common problem for type 1 sugar addicts. Indigestion can be aggravated by the overuse of antacids. Contrary to popular belief, the problem isn't that you make too much stomach acid, but rather that you make too little.

Antacids just exacerbate this problem and can even be addictive. In addition to blocking the absorption of vitamin B_{12} and many other nutrients from your food, acid blocker medications can decrease absorption of thyroid hormone, which further fuels sugar cravings.

Constipation can also be an issue. When you don't eat foods with fiber and load up on sugar instead, the "transit time" that food is in your digestive system increases; food tends to putrefy in the digestive tract, releasing toxins. You get brain fog and feel sluggish and achy. In the extreme, chronic fatigue syndrome and fibromyalgia may develop.

SLEEP DEPRIVATION IN TYPE 1 SUGAR ADDICTS

Insomnia is a common problem for type 1 sugar addicts. Obviously, if you don't get enough sleep, you won't have much energy—and you'll be more likely to reach for energy drinks to fuel your sugar addiction during the day. Your punishing schedule leaves you little time for sleep and makes it hard for you to fall asleep. Many of you average only six hours of sleep a night.

Sleep is critical for many functions. It recharges your batteries, helps tissues repair, and enables you to produce growth hormone. Without enough growth hormone, you will age more rapidly and may develop chronic achiness and pain.

Sleep also regulates the production of ghrelin and leptin—the appetite-controlling hormones—so you are more likely to reach for that sugary drink. In fact, a six-year-long study of 276 adults conducted by researchers at Laval University in Quebec City, Quebec, found that sleeping fewer than seven hours a night increases your risk of obesity by 30 percent and causes an average weight gain of 5 pounds (23 kg).

Fortunately, natural remedies can help most people with insomnia. In part II, you will learn about the best natural and prescription therapies so you can get eight hours of solid sleep a night.

Summary: Key Features of the Type 1 Sugar Addict

- Type 1 sugar addicts often have type A personalities. You strive for perfection in whatever you do.

- Many type 1 sugar addicts are hooked on energy drinks, coffee, and caffeinated sodas.

- Energy drinks, coffee, and caffeinated sodas give you a temporary boost, but leave you feeling even more tired.

- Using caffeine and sugar to boost energy artificially can lead to all sorts of health problems, including an impaired immune system, sleep disorders, headaches, high blood pressure, chronic fatigue syndrome, and fibromyalgia.

- You can feel better by following the SHINE Protocol (see chapter 6).

2

TYPE 2 SUGAR ADDICTION: FEED ME NOW OR I'LL KILL YOU

When life's stress has exhausted your adrenal glands

The type 2 sugar addict is constantly reacting to stressful stimuli in the environment, which activates the adrenal glands to produce the stress-handler hormones cortisol and epinephrine (adrenaline). When your adrenals become overtaxed by the constant tension of modern life and don't respond by giving you a kick of energy, you may reach for sugar to "pump them up." But this effect is short-lived, followed by a drop in blood sugar known as hypoglycemia. Starved of glucose (its food), your brain feels like it's suffocating. You become anxious, jittery, and light-headed. You need to eat *now*. You can't wait. And if you don't eat—preferably something sweet—the symptoms just get worse.

TAKE THIS QUIZ

Your total score will tell you whether you fit the type 2 profile. Do you?

____	Do you find that you are always thirsty and have to urinate frequently? (10 points)
____	Do you get recurrent sore throats and swollen glands? (10 points)
____	Is life a crisis to you? (15 points)
____	Do you enjoy the rush of energy you feel when you are in a crisis? (15 points)
✗	When you are stressed out, does your energy take a nosedive? (15 points)
____	Do you sometimes get dizzy when you stand? (15 points)
____	Do you have chronic severe exhaustion, chronic fatigue syndrome, or fibromyalgia, which followed an acute infection or an incident of extreme stress? (25 points)
____	Are you very irritable when hungry? Do you get a "Feed me *now* or I'll kill you" feeling? (35 points)
____	Your total score

SCORE	
0–24:	You are probably a type B "low-key" person with healthy adrenals.
25–49:	You are developing early stages of adrenal fatigue.
50–75:	This suggests moderate adrenal exhaustion, and your body is crying out for help.
Over 75:	You are suffering from severe adrenal exhaustion and likely are feeling awful overall.

WHAT DOES A TYPICAL TYPE 2 SUGAR ADDICT LOOK LIKE?

If you are a type 2 sugar addict, you feel like you are always in crisis. You don't act, you react, which sets off a chain of events guaranteed to leave you stressed out. You are a master at making mountains out of molehills because your distorted thinking and behavior change a small event into a big problem. When you feel burned out by stress, you reach for sugar.

You are also often the "go-to" person when problems arise. It's admirable to help others, but type 2 sugar addicts are often people pleasers who routinely put others' needs before their own. Other people's approval is necessary so you can feel good about yourself, and you won't rest until their problems are solved. But instead of taking a break when you feel fatigued, you snack on sugar.

Type 2 sugar addicts are often stressed out women, juggling their roles as wives and mothers with demanding jobs outside their homes. You are always on the run: to soccer practice, to ballet class, to work, and home again. You are exhausted, but you can't seem to stop. When you crash, you reach for a sugar fix to artificially pump up your tired adrenal glands, which fuels your sugar addiction.

Initially, though, this approach seems to work, and even though your adrenals are taxed by stress, you may still feel pretty good. That's because you've become an adrenaline junkie and the rush keeps you on an "energy high."

Eventually, this backfires. As you repeatedly "use" sugar to get an energy boost, your blood sugar dips even lower, and that drives the adrenals to work even harder. Over time, the adrenal glands may become bigger, just as muscles do when you work out. Ultimately, however, your adrenals become exhausted.

You may find it difficult to get out of bed in the morning. You might suffer from chronic sore throats and recurrent swollen glands in your neck. You get sick more often and have difficulty recovering. You may have low blood pressure and feel dizzy upon standing. You might even develop chronic fatigue syndrome.

If you are a type 2 sugar addict, you may find that you can no longer fit into your skinny jeans. That's because every time the adrenals kick in, insulin is released, telling the body to store more fat. In two of our studies at the Annapolis Chronic Fatigue and Fibromyalgia Research Center, people with chronic fatigue syndrome or fibromyalgia, with associated adrenal fatigue, had an average weight gain of 32.5 pounds (15 kg).

The key sign of adrenal fatigue, however, is hypoglycemia, or low blood sugar. This condition can make you irritable when you're hungry. You feel like you need something to eat right *now*! Usually that something is sugar.

THE ROLLER COASTER RIDE OF HYPOGLYCEMIA

When you eat sugar, your blood glucose rises sharply. Your body then releases high amounts of insulin, causing your sugar to plummet quickly. Low blood sugar creates a sugar craving and puts you on an emotional (and blood sugar) roller coaster.

Having large amounts of sugar and white flour in the diet is a fairly new phenomenon in human history. In the past, we ate whole and unprocessed foods that took a few hours to slowly digest, releasing a steady stream of sugar into your blood during that time.

The Adrenal Glands and Blood Sugar

The adrenal glands, controlled by the pituitary, are located on either side of your kidneys and maintain stable blood sugar levels by producing cortisol, which triggers the manufacture of insulin. But when you are under stress (in a fight or flight situation), the glands produce adrenaline or epinephrine, which increases your blood sugar, heart rate, and pulse to prepare you for action. Without enough cortisol and in turn, insulin, to handle the spike, your blood sugar rapidly drops during stress and your brain feels like you're drowning.

You do need a normal amount of adrenaline on a day-to-day basis. The adrenal glands help maintain normal energy levels for balancing the immune system, maintaining healthy blood pressure, and producing other hormones, including dehydroepiandrosterone sulfate (DHEA, the "fountain of youth hormone"), aldosterone (which maintains proper salt and water levels in the body), and even some of your testosterone.

For example, when you eat a turkey and cheese sandwich on whole wheat bread (something with a low glycemic index), it takes a few hours for your body to digest it, and your blood sugar rises slowly. (We'll talk more about the glycemic index later.) Insulin is steadily released to help unlock the door to the cells, allowing sugar or glucose to leave your bloodstream and enter the cells to be burned as fuel. Blood sugar and insulin levels both go down gradually after a few hours, and you have a healthy pattern of blood sugar rise and fall.

But when your adrenal glands are exhausted, you are more likely to consume sugar in large quantities in an attempt to get the energy you need. Maybe you drink a 12-ounce (355 ml) can of soda that contains *10* teaspoons (40 g) of sugar. When the sugar hits your system, your blood sugar skyrockets and your body dramatically increases insulin production to process the sugar out of the bloodstream into the cells. This causes a steep dip in blood sugar levels, which results in hypoglycemia.

Hypoglycemia stimulates a craving for sugar, along with anxiety and irritability. But every time you eat that candy bar or gulp that soda, you put your body under more stress and exacerbate your sugar addiction.

THE PRICE TYPE 2 SUGAR ADDICTS PAY OVER TIME

Overproduction of cortisol, which happens when you are excessively stressed out, suppresses immune function. But when the adrenals are finally exhausted, too little cortisol causes immune dysfunction as well and can increase sugar cravings. The long-term consequences can be severe:

- Chronic fatigue syndrome and fibromyalgia are characterized by insomnia despite exhaustion because your adrenal glands lose their ability for self-regulation. Cortisol levels are low during the day, causing fatigue and irritability. At night, as cortisol levels rise too high, insomnia occurs. Low blood sugar can also throw your muscles into spasm, causing chronic pain.

- Immune function also suffers when cortisol levels drop. The result is an increase in autoimmune diseases (e.g., lupus). This also makes you more prone to catching colds and flu.

- Excess cortisol can cause elevated blood sugar and diabetes. It directly increases blood pressure (hypertension), can lead to loss of bone strength (osteoporosis), and produces weight gain (sometimes massive) from the elevated insulin levels.

Many people who have low adrenal problems also have low thyroid function. Because blood tests are not reliable, your doctor will need to diagnose you according to your symptoms, which include fatigue, aches and pains, weight gain, and cold intolerance. It's important to treat both of these conditions at once. If you treat a low thyroid without treating the adrenals, you actually stress the adrenals and can make your symptoms worse. You'll find more information about treating hypothyroidism in part III.

The Adrenal Glands and Blood Sugar

- When your adrenals become overtaxed by stress, you reach for sugar to "pump them up." This can lead to sugar addiction.

- Type 2 sugar addicts suffer from adrenal exhaustion, a common condition that affects millions of Americans, especially women.

- Type 2 sugar addicts have low blood sugar or hypoglycemia.

- If untreated and severe, the long-term consequences of adrenal fatigue can result in chronic fatigue and fibromyalgia, immune dysfunction, diabetes, high blood pressure, osteoporosis, and obesity.

- Type 2 sugar addicts may also have hypothyroidism.

- You can break your sugar addiction by changing your diet and treating adrenal fatigue with bio-identical cortisol taken in tiny (physiological) amounts. You will also need to take vitamin C, high dose pantothenic acid (vitamin B_5), licorice, and chromium. You'll need to learn how to handle stress better, too. (See chapter 7.)

CHAPTER

3

TYPE 3 SUGAR ADDICTION: THE HAPPY HO-HO HUNTER

Sugar cravings caused by yeast/candida overgrowth

A type 3 sugar addict needs sugar fixes regularly. From morning to night, the type 3 sugar addict noshes on donuts, Danish, cookies, cake, Ho-Hos, and other sweets. Without knowing it, however, when you feed yourself sugar, you are also feeding the yeast in your body. No, we're not talking about the type that you use to make bread rise. We're talking *Candida albicans*, the type that grows in your digestive system from fermenting sugar and carbs. When yeast ferments hops to make beer, that's a good thing. When it uses your gut as a fermentation tank, though, the result is pretty toxic. And it sends your sugar addiction spiraling out of control.

TAKE THIS QUIZ

Your total score will tell you whether you fit the type 3 profile. Do you?

___	Do you have chronic nasal congestion or sinusitis? (50 points)
✗	Do you have spastic colon or irritable bowel syndrome (gas, bloating, and diarrhea and/or constipation)? (50 points)
___	Have you been treated for acne with tetracycline, erythromycin, or any other antibiotic for one month or longer? (50 points)
___	Have you taken antibiotics for any type of infection for more than two consecutive months or shorter courses more than three times in a twelve-month period? (20 points)
6	Have you taken an antibiotic—even for a single course? (6 points)
___	Do you have chronic fatigue syndrome or fibromyalgia? (50 points)
___	Have you had prostatitis or chronic yeast vaginitis? (25 points)
5	Have you been pregnant? (5 points)
___	Have you taken birth control pills? (10 points)
___	Have you taken corticosteroids, such as Prednisone, for over a month? (15 points)
10	When you are exposed to perfumes, insecticides, or other odors or chemicals, do you develop wheezing, burning eyes, or any other distress? (10 points)
10	Are your symptoms worse on damp or humid days or in moldy places? (10 points)
___	Have you had a fungal infection, such as jock itch, athlete's foot, or a nail or skin infection, that was difficult to treat? (20 points)
___	Do you have postnasal drip or clear your throat a lot? (20 points)
20	Do you crave sugar or breads? (20 points)
20	Do you have food allergies? (20 points)
72	Your total score

Candida Yeast grows from fermenting Sugar & Carb

SCORE

If your total is 70 or higher, you likely have a yeast/candida overgrowth and need the treatment outlined in chapter 8.

WHAT DOES A TYPE 3 SUGAR ADDICT LOOK LIKE?

Your life revolves around sugar. Someone mentions sweets and your eyes light up. You eat sugar all day long, starting with a breakfast of coffee and a sweet Danish or yummy donut. This sugar-laden feast just gears you up to want more. By mid-morning you reach for a candy bar from the vending machine. Lunch is a sandwich on white bread (which quickly converts to glucose: sugar) washed down with a large soft drink. By mid-afternoon, you need a snack and reach for cookies, Twinkies, or a Ho-Ho, and don't forget a bedtime snack! You constantly crave sugar and make sure you always have cookies, cake, and other sweets in your kitchen, office, purse, and car. It's not unusual to see you at the local convenience store in the middle of the night getting your fix.

But the price of overindulging in sweets is high. A type 3 sugar addict often feels tired; you may even have chronic fatigue syndrome and fibromyalgia. It doesn't stop there. Yeast overgrowth fueled by sugar can cause numerous other health problems, like sinusitis or postnasal drip. When this happens, you'll see the doctor for antibiotics to treat what you think is a sinus infection. You may also have problems with your digestion, such as gas, bloating, diarrhea and/or constipation, and irritable bowel syndrome. Poor eating habits and eating sugar-laden foods can also mean that you are overweight or obese. You may even be allergic to these foods, although you don't realize it. More about this later.

THE ROLE OF YEAST IN SUGAR ADDICTION

Why does sugar cause so many problems? Sugar and yeast have a symbiotic relationship. In fact, yeast grow from the fermenting sugars in your body. Yeast can also make you feel like you have no will power, triggering your sugar cravings by releasing a certain chemical, so you'll feed them their favorite food. Smart, huh? So whenever you eat sweets, you're feeding the yeast as well. Although science has not yet tracked down the chemical that triggers the sugar cravings, experience with many thousands of patients shows that their sugar cravings decrease dramatically after the yeast have been killed off.

Here's how this vicious cycle works. The yeast in your gut cause sugar cravings, driving you to eat more sugar, which makes your yeast grow and multiply, which in turn makes you crave more sugar. The result? A yeast overgrowth—billions of baby yeast, fungi, or candida. If you are a type 3 sugar addict trapped in this cycle, you know how awful it can be.

To compound the problem, yeast are really *big*. If, for example, a virus is the size of a ballpoint pen tip and bacteria are the size of a sofa, yeast can be the size of your whole living room. Because of their sheer size, yeast overgrowth causes a huge challenge for your immune system. When yeast turns into long threads called mycelia that grow through the abdominal wall, it makes the problem of sugar craving even worse.

The abdominal wall is the main barrier, along with your skin, that determines what stays outside of your body. To act as a good gatekeeper, the lining of your intestines needs to be intact and whole. But when mycelia permeate the abdominal wall, you end up with "leaky gut syndrome." This means instead of absorbing digested food, you absorb partially digested chunks of protein before they've been reduced to individual amino acids that the body can utilize. Unfortunately, these chunks of protein can then trigger many kinds of allergic and other problematic reactions.

For example, partially digested protein puts your immune system on high alert because the body treats it as an outside invader. The question the immune system asks as it defends the body is "Are you self or other?" If it recognizes the undigested protein as being part of you, it lets it pass. But if it thinks that undigested protein is "other," it goes into action, finishing off the job of digesting your food, and stressing it even further by pushing it into overdrive. It can also trigger allergies to certain foods which we discuss below. The result? You feel tired—and reach for more sugar to artificially boost your energy.

How Antibiotic Abuse Contributes to the Yeast-Sugar Cycle

Yeast overgrowth can also be exacerbated by the overuse of antibiotics to treat the chronic sinus, bladder, prostate, and respiratory infections—infections that the yeast actually triggered. Antibiotics kill harmful bacteria that cause infections, but also wipe out the "good" bacteria—allowing the yeast to flourish.

Good bacteria or flora are essential for your health. They help digest your food, play a role in nutrition, and prevent the overgrowth of "bad" bacteria or infections in your body. In fact, there are normally more healthy bacteria in your colon (about 10 trillion) than there are cells in your body. One of their critical jobs is preventing yeast from overgrowing and causing problems.

When you take antibiotics, which kill off the bacteria but not the yeast, the yeast have no competition. Now they can grow unchecked. This makes sugar cravings much worse.

Other Factors That Exacerbate the Yeast-Sugar Problem

Frequently popping antacids can also cause yeast overgrowth and worsen sugar cravings. Antacids turn off the stomach acid that usually kills the yeast in the food we eat. Using steroids like Prednisone (for asthma or other inflammation) suppresses your immune system, too, and allows yeast to grow.

If you don't get enough sleep, you may fuel yeast overgrowth and sugar cravings as well. Sleep is absolutely essential for a healthy immune system. If your immune system doesn't work properly, you can't get rid of infections.

Feeling stressed? Stress can also play a role in yeast overgrowth. That's because when you are stressed, your body secretes cortisol (see chapter 2). Chronic high levels of cortisol suppress your immune system and allow the yeast to run wild, making sugar cravings constant.

The Link between Yeast Overgrowth and Food Allergies

A yeast overgrowth can also cause food allergies. The most common food allergies are to wheat, milk, chocolate, citrus, and eggs. Often, what we are allergic to we crave the most. The more you eat of something, the more allergic you become, because your immune system sees more of the proteins in those foods. If you are allergic to chocolate, for example, you want to eat it all the more. More sugar, more yeast. More yeast, more allergies. That's why it's sometimes necessary to treat food allergies in conjunction with yeast overgrowth. (We'll talk more about this in chapter 8.)

Different foods contain different proteins. When some food proteins are only partially broken down during digestion, they can mimic various hormones and neurotransmitters in the body. Wheat, for example, contains gluten, which has protein chunks that mimic endorphin. Although we think of endorphin as the "happy hormone" that causes the "runner's high," when it gets into the bloodstream and into the brain where it doesn't belong, it can lead to inflammation. Schizophrenia, for instance, has been associated with wheat and milk allergies, and patients improve much more quickly when they avoid wheat and milk.

Allergies can also cause emotional problems, such as mood shifts, anxiety, and depression. When you feel anxious, depressed, or emotionally upset, you're more likely to reach for something sweet to eat—comfort foods like cookies and ice cream are favorites. And the cycle continues.

THE PRICE TYPE 3 SUGAR ADDICTS PAY OVER TIME

In addition to causing allergies, yeast overgrowth can lead to chronic conditions for type 3 sugar addicts, such as chronic fatigue syndrome (CFS), fibromyalgia, and immune dysfunction. Our research at the Annapolis Chronic Fatigue and Fibromyalgia Research Center shows that if you have CFS, you improve when you eliminate the yeast. Research by Birgitta Evengård, MD, PhD, a specialist in infectious diseases and clinical immunology at Huddinge University Hospital and an associate professor and lecturer at Karolinska Institute in Stockholm, Sweden, has even found higher bowel candida levels to be present during CFS flare-ups.

Although there is no test to distinguish fungal overgrowth from normal fungal levels, you can diagnose overgrowth by symptoms, such as the allergies we just discussed, nasal congestion or sinusitis, spastic colon, unusual rashes, and food allergies. Holistic doctors often target yeast in people who have these symptoms and achieve very positive results. In part III, you'll find out more about treatments for several common conditions, including sinusitis and spastic colon.

Summary: Key Features of the Type 3 Sugar Addict

1. Yeast overgrowth occurs largely because of excessive sugar in your diet.

2. Sugar cravings are caused by yeast, and the yeast eat sugar to multiply.

3. Excessive use of antibiotics and steroids exacerbate yeast overgrowth.

4. Spastic colon and sinusitis are two common problems largely caused by yeast; they often go away when the yeast overgrowth is treated.

5. Using Dr. Doris Rapp's Elimination Diet and adding herbs, antifungals, and probiotics can help break your sugar addiction (see chapter 8).

CHAPTER

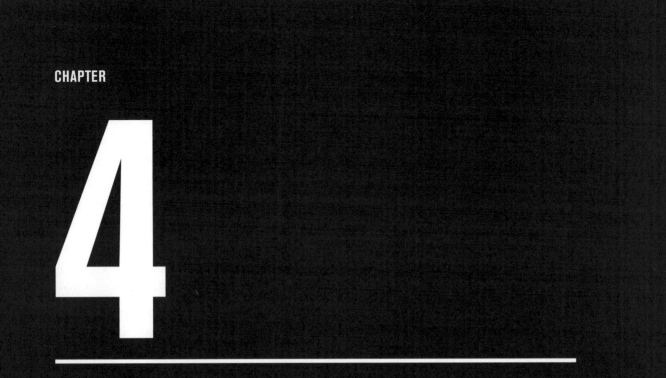

4

TYPE 4 SUGAR ADDICTION: DEPRESSED AND CRAVING CARBS: *Sugar cravings caused by your period, menopause, or andropause*

Hormones are a critical part of your body's communication and control system. For this reason, hormone deficiencies—or even imbalances—can wreak havoc with your physical and emotional well-being. If you have a deficiency of estrogen, progesterone, and/or testosterone (if you're a woman) or testosterone (if you're a man), you're likely to crave sugar. That's because when these hormone levels are low, you become sad, even depressed. You start craving sugar as your body tries to raise its level of serotonin, "the happiness molecule." Anxiety can also occur from low progesterone, causing a drop in your body's GABA (gamma-aminobutyric acid) or "natural Valium" levels. This can produce adrenal fatigue and type 2 sugar cravings (see chapters 2 and 6). In some cases, your sugar cravings may be due to insulin resistance or diabetes.

TAKE THIS QUIZ

Your total score will tell you whether you fit the type 4 profile. Do you?

Women

PMS	
____	Do you have a history of PMS (premenstrual syndrome)? (30 points)
Or, in the week before your period, do you have increased and severe:	
____	Irritability? (15 points)
15	Anxiety? (15 points)
15	Unhappiness or depression? (15 points)
15	Bloating? (15 points)
45	Your total score

If you scored 30 or higher, read the section on PMS below.

MENOPAUSE OR PERIMENOPAUSE	
Are you older than thirty-eight or have you had a hysterectomy or ovarian surgery? If so:	
25	Do you have decreased vaginal lubrication? (25 points)
15	Do you have decreased sex drive (libido)? (15 points)
____	Have you had periods been getting irregular or changing in other ways? (15 points)
In the week before and around your period, do you experience noticeably worse:	
____	Insomnia? (15 points)
____	Headaches? (15 points)
____	Fatigue? (15 points)
____	Hot flashes or sweats? (20 points)
40	Your total score

If you scored 30 or higher, you likely have symptoms from estrogen or progesterone deficiency; read the section on perimenopause and menopause below.

Are you older than forty-seven and have your periods stopped or have you had a hysterectomy? If so, do you have:	
____	Depression? (15 points)
____	Vaginal dryness? (15 points)
____	Fatigue? (15 points)
____	Insomnia? (15 points)
____	Loss of libido? (15 points)
____	Your total score

If you scored 30 or higher, you likely have symptoms from hormone deficiency associated with menopause; read the section on perimenopause and menopause below.

Men

____	Are you older than forty-five? (15 points)
____	Do you have decreased libido? (20 points)
____	Do you have erectile dysfunction or decrease in erections? (20 points)
____	Do you have hypertension? (20 points)
____	Do you have diabetes? (20 points)
____	Do you have high cholesterol? (20 points)
____	Are you overweight with a "spare tire" around your waist? (20 points)
____	Your total score

If you scored 50 or higher, these symptoms may be the result of an inadequate testosterone level. Ignore the "normal range" for testosterone levels on the lab result (even if your doctor uses it) and instead use the ranges we supply in chapter 9.

WHAT DOES A TYPE 4 SUGAR ADDICT LOOK LIKE?

Thanks to hormonal fluctuations, women can have more difficulty controlling their emotions at certain times during their menstrual cycle. You may feel tired, irritable, and cranky—and you crave sugar. If you are in perimenopause or menopause, you have hot flashes, fatigue, mood swings, headaches, and intense sugar cravings when estrogen, progesterone, and even testosterone levels plummet during the four to seven days around your period. If you are a man older than forty-five, you may experience a hormonal imbalance called andropause, when testosterone levels decline, causing you to crave sugar. Sound like you? Then, you're probably a type 4 sugar addict.

THE ROLE OF INSULIN IN SUGAR REGULATION

Insulin is the hormone that regulates blood sugar. Just as your car burns gasoline, your body burns sugar for fuel—and the sugar must be made available to cells in just the right amounts. Too much sugar and you flood the system, stressing your body and causing it to make excess insulin. This drives down your blood sugar, leaving you irritable and anxious, and then exhausted and craving sugar.

Insulin acts like the key that opens the door to your cellular furnaces, so that sugar can get into your cells from your bloodstream to be burned as fuel. When the system is working properly, your body actually makes the sugar needed for fuel (usually from protein and complex carbohydrates), burning calories and regulating hunger. You feel energetic, and you burn calories while staying slim and trim.

When you have insulin resistance, however, the key that opens the "furnace doors" to your cells doesn't work. Instead, sugar builds up in your blood. Meanwhile, your cells are starved for sugar to make energy and cry out for more sugar. Because the sugar can't get into your cells to be burned for fuel, you may feel tired and depressed—and find yourself craving sugar. The sugar you eat does not help—it just triggers your body to make more insulin—and you feel exhausted and moody. At the same time, blood sugar, cholesterol, and triglyceride (blood fat) levels climb higher and higher. When severe, it is the most common cause of adult diabetes.

You may also gain weight. The sugar can't be burned for fuel, so it has to go somewhere. Usually it gets turned into fat. In women, excess insulin levels pack fat onto your hips, thighs, and butt. In men, the fat gets stashed around your waist, creating that "spare tire" look.

In men, low testosterone (even if your blood levels are technically "normal") is a major cause of insulin resistance. The testosterone deficiency can then cause high cholesterol, high blood pressure, depression, osteoporosis, and obesity in addition to diabetes and heart disease.

Paradoxically, in women, an elevated testosterone level, as can be seen in polycystic ovarian syndrome, can also cause insulin resistance. Low estrogen and menopause have also been associated with insulin resistance (although it's less common than andropause-related insulin resistance in men). Using synthetic progesterone (i.e., Provera) to treat menopause can also worsen insulin resistance. A healthier approach? Natural alternatives, such as edamame (soybean pods), black cohosh (Remifemin), or bio-identical hormones, which you'll learn more about in chapter 9.

SUGAR CRAVINGS LINKED WITH PMS

PMS is a mix of symptoms, including irritability and sugar cravings, that worsen around a woman's menstrual cycle. The cause of PMS is controversial, but holistic doctors have found that PMS is usually associated with inadequate progesterone and prostaglandin levels—two hormones that are critical to how you feel.

Normally, your estrogen and progesterone levels fluctuate throughout the month to enable pregnancy to occur. These two hormones rise in the first two weeks of the cycle (the follicular phase) and dip during ovulation. Because of this ovulatory dip, it's common for women to experience estrogen-related migraines, heart palpitations, and anxiety attacks during ovulation at the midpoint of the menstrual cycle.

After ovulation, estrogen and progesterone levels rise again and these symptoms are ameliorated. During your period, estrogen and progesterone levels drop to their lowest levels (similar to what happens in menopause), resulting in the symptoms of estrogen and progesterone deficiency—and sugar cravings.

PMS is predominately a progesterone deficiency. Progesterone stimulates production of the brain chemical called GABA (gamma-aminobutyric acid), which acts as your body's "natural Valium" to calm you and help you sleep. When progesterone is too low, you feel anxious and irritable and may experience insomnia. When progesterone is too high, you may feel depressed. Progesterone deficiency often triggers sugar cravings and causes you to reach for sugar to ease the symptoms. It works, initially. Unfortunately, after the "sugar high" wears off, your blood sugar plummets, leaving you feeling even more anxious and hyper.

Do You Have PMS?

To determine whether you have PMS, it can be helpful to keep a mood diary for several months. Compare the intensity of your emotional symptoms and sugar cravings on days five through ten of your cycle (day one is the first day of your period) to the six-day interval before the onset of menses. To qualify as PMS, the intensity of your symptoms will usually increase by at least 30 percent in the six days before menstruation. This pattern must be documented for at least two consecutive cycles.

Once you realize that your moods are associated with changes in your hormones around your period, you and the people close to you can better understand and cope with the symptoms. In addition, the treatments we recommend in chapter 9 can help stabilize your emotions and sugar cravings.

SUGAR CRAVINGS LINKED WITH PERIMENOPAUSE AND MENOPAUSE

During menopause, the production of estrogen and progesterone decline as the ovaries wear out. This decline impacts the body profoundly. This is not a sudden event, but rather occurs gradually over a period of five to twelve years, known as perimenopause. Menopause and perimenopause can trigger symptoms of fatigue and depression, which many women try to treat by eating sugar. Low estrogen in menopause also causes brain fog, fatigue, achiness, headache/migraine, lower libido, insomnia, and hot flashes. This can be especially prominent in people who have chronic fatigue and fibromyalgia. The low progesterone levels also cause insomnia and anxiety. Menopause symptoms include the following:

- Menstrual cycles become irregular (becoming either heavier or lighter)

- Weight gain may occur

- Fatigue

- Low libido

- Worsening headaches

- Brain fog

- Mood swings, irritability, or feelings of depression

Although testosterone deficiency is a larger problem in men, it also is a significant issue for women. Even though a woman's testosterone levels do not drop as quickly as her estrogen and progesterone levels do during menopause (because the adrenal glands make half of a woman's testosterone), most menopausal women are testosterone deficient—despite the testosterone being too high relative to the low estrogen. This low testosterone can also contribute to loss of libido as well as muscle wasting, depression, and fatigue, which can lead to sugar cravings. Once the estrogen and progesterone deficiencies have been corrected, then a very low dose of natural bio-identical testosterone can also be safely added to help restore libido and energy. You can learn more about this in chapter 9.

Many conventional doctors do not diagnose menopause until there is total failure of your ovaries and total cessation of your periods. This means that you must be estrogen deficient for five to twelve years before a doctor will diagnose menopause and consider support with estrogen. We'll also talk more about this in chapter 9.

Using Sugar to Raise Serotonin and Feel Better

Low estrogen levels in PMS, perimenopause, and menopause affect the production of the "happiness molecule" serotonin as well as other brain chemicals (neurotransmitters) that, when deficient, can trigger depression and sugar cravings. Serotonin also is critical for sleep and curbing appetite (it gives a sense of fullness).

Serotonin is produced from the amino acid (protein) called tryptophan, which requires vitamin B_6 (pyridoxine) and magnesium to be converted into serotonin. Other B vitamins are also essential for emotional health. For example, if there is a deficiency of vitamin B_3 (niacin), the body will use dietary tryptophan to synthesize niacin.

In the short term, eating sugar raises serotonin levels and makes you feel happier. This occurs because as the sugar raises insulin, the insulin drives many amino acids (proteins) into your muscles, but not tryptophan, leaving more tryptophan free to go into your brain to make serotonin.

Unfortunately, as insulin resistance occurs, this antidepressant and the feel-good benefits of sugar decrease. In fact, the insulin resistance can then cause a drop in serotonin levels in the brain, so once again eating sugar becomes counterproductive. So although eating something sweet may initially make you feel better, it leads to even worse blood sugar fluctuations, exacerbation of your symptoms, and ultimately sugar addiction.

SUGAR CRAVINGS LINKED WITH ANDROPAUSE

In men, testosterone deficiency associated with andropause, or male menopause, can also cause sugar cravings along with insulin resistance and fatigue. Other problems caused by testosterone deficiency in men include depression, decreased libido, decreased erectile function, loss of drive and stamina, osteoporosis, high blood pressure, weight gain, diabetes, and high cholesterol. Supplementation with bio-identical natural testosterone can decrease and sometimes eliminate metabolic syndrome (high blood pressure, diabetes, and high cholesterol), even in men with borderline low but technically "normal" levels of testosterone.

Perhaps you've heard that testosterone may increase the risk of prostate cancer and other problems. Numerous studies have shown that this is not the case. (See chapter 8.) The controversy surrounding the use of dangerous synthetic hormones in both women and bodybuilders has resulted in the elimination of much of the National Institutes of Health funding for testosterone use in males. On the positive side, now that new expensive prescription testosterone creams are available for men, drug companies are pouring money into this research.

Summary: Key Features of the Type 4 Sugar Addict

1. Deficiency of estrogen, progesterone, and/or testosterone in women can lead to sugar addiction because of insulin resistance, anxiety, and depression.

2. Testosterone deficiency in men can lead to sugar addiction because of insulin resistance, diabetes, and depression.

3. Using bio-identical hormones and/or other natural remedies such as herbs can help you break your sugar addiction.

PART 2

THE SOLUTION

Now that you've figured out which type of sugar addict you are, it's time to start fixing the problem. Chances are, you're feeling a bit overwhelmed. That's okay. Just take a nice deep breath and relax. This is a journey, not a quick jaunt. Our intention in part II is to help you do the following:

1. Eliminate the underlying problems that are driving your sugar addiction. This will make it much easier for you to give up excess sugar and stay off it.

2. Enjoy sweets in moderation, for example, as dessert or an occasional snack.

3. Eliminate the physical and psychological problems caused by sugar addiction, so you can feel great.

CHAPTER

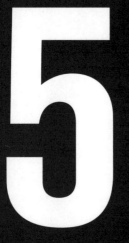

HEALING PRACTICES FOR ALL SUGAR ADDICTS

In this section, you'll learn all about commonsense practices that will help all four types of sugar addicts to begin the process of kicking their addiction. In the four chapters that follow, you'll learn how to use the treatment protocol for your specific sugar addiction type(s), as determined in part I. Pleasure is good, and our goal is to show you how to enjoy what you eat while staying healthy. In short, we're going to teach you how to "have your cake and eat it, too."

CUT OUT SUGAR

The first step in breaking your addiction is to change the way you eat. The most important thing, of course, is to stop eating sugar. Eating sugar just fans the fires of your addiction and keeps you stuck in a vicious cycle. As with any addiction, you have to cut out the addictive substance before you can begin healing the problem. You don't have to do it all at once or cut out all of the sugar. Start simply by getting rid of high-sugar foods in your diet, including fast food, processed food, sodas, and fruit drinks.

Read the labels. Sugar has many other names. Besides those ending in "ose," such as maltose or sucrose, other names for sugar include high fructose corn syrup, molasses, cane sugar, corn sweetener, raw sugar, syrup, honey, or fruit juice concentrates. As a rule of thumb, don't eat anything that lists sugar in any form (sugar, sucrose, glucose, fructose, or corn syrup) as one of the top three ingredients on the label. In addition, you'll also want to avoid the white flour found in many breads and pasta because your body rapidly converts this into sugar, giving you a sugar high and then a low. Though it's an acquired taste (like beer), you'll find, over time, that whole grain breads taste much better. Enjoy them in moderation.

Avoid added sugars. Added sugars are sugars and syrups put in foods during preparation or processing. The major sources of added sugars are soda, candy, cakes, cup cakes, cookies, pies, fruit drinks, desserts, various milk products (such as ice cream and yogurt), and grains like cereal and waffles.

To find out if a particular food has added sugars, check the Nutrition Facts panel. The line for sugars contains both the natural sugars and the added types of sugars as total grams of sugar. There are four calories in each gram, so if a product has 15 grams of sugar per serving, that's 60 calories from sugar. According to the American Heart Association, women should consume no more than 100 calories per day from added sugars, while men should eat or drink no more than 150 calories per day.

A more intuitive and simple approach is to divide the number of grams of sugar by four to determine how many teaspoons of sugar there are per serving.

Labeling Added Sugars

For the first time in two decades, on February, 27, 2014, the Food and Drug Administration proposed an overhaul to all nutrition labels on packaged foods. Soon, consumers will know just how much sugar has been added by manufacturers. Added sugars will be noted on the nutrition facts panel along with portion sizes and total nutrition information for multiple servings instead of naturally-occurring and added sugars combined into a single listing of "total sugars."

WITHDRAWAL FROM SUGAR ADDICTION

As you change your diet and cut out sugar, don't be surprised if you experience withdrawal symptoms such as moodiness and irritability. This is even more likely if you are trying to kick caffeine at the same time. The good news is that it will pass in seven to ten days and often even quicker when you treat the issues underlying your specific sugar addiction type. Although withdrawal can be a bit uncomfortable for some people, most of you won't find it a significant problem, especially if you apply the sugar addiction treatments we'll discuss here in part II.

If withdrawal symptoms are an issue, reduce your sugar and caffeine intake more gradually. Allow yourself a healthy snack of fruit and even a few pieces of the best-tasting dark chocolate you can find. This will make it easier for you to stick with the program.

SUGAR SUBSTITUTES

Sugar substitutes can give you some of the pleasure of sugar without the side effects. Today, there are more choices than ever before. Keep in mind though that some substitutes are healthy and some aren't. Let's take a look at some of the most common substitutes.

Stevia

This excellent sugar substitute is safe, healthy, and natural. Used for many decades, it has recently been approved by the FDA for use in food processing. Therefore, more and more foods and even sodas that include this healthy sugar substitute will soon be available.

Stevia comes from leaves of the stevia plant, an herb in the chrysanthemum family. It grows wild as a small shrub in parts of Paraguay and Brazil. The leaves contain an extract (called a stevioside) that may be 200 to 300 times as sweet as sugar. This extract is safe and contains no calories. It can be used in cooking and as an excellent overall sugar substitute. It is even safe for diabetics.

Keep in mind, however, that unless stevia is properly filtered it will leave a bitter or licorice aftertaste. If you get a brand that does not taste good, it was not properly filtered. Simply switch brands. A good brand is Body Ecology. It comes as a clear liquid in a dropper bottle. Another good brand is Stevita, which can be found in many health food stores.

Sugar Alcohols

These are also safe and healthy sugar substitutes. In sugar alcohols, the sugar has been converted through a natural fermenting process to resemble alcohol—but not the form that gets you drunk. It still tastes sweet but is not absorbed into your body, so it does not cause the problems sugar does. The most common one is the maltitol used in sugar-free chocolates. The only downside of most of the sugar alcohols is that they can have a laxative effect, causing gas and loose stools in some people. If this occurs and is problematic, simply eat less of it.

Other sugar alcohols include inositol, which is helpful for anxiety (and improves bone density in people with osteoporosis), and most other substances ending in the letters ol.

Erythritol

Erythritol is an excellent alternative for those who can't tolerate the other sugar alcohols. It provides all of the benefits of sugar alcohols without the gas or bloating. It is absorbed by the body, but is then quickly eliminated in the urine. Erythritol is not metabolized in your body and is basically inert (it does nothing, good or bad). Although it is fifteen times as sweet as sugar, it's considered by many to have zero calories.

Erythritol's popularity is growing, and it will become even more readily available as Truvia and PureVia (which are mixes of erythritol and stevia) go mainstream. Truvia, developed by Cargill, is being added to a line of Coca-Cola and Sprite products and Glaceau vitamin water.

Chemical Sweeteners

Each of the three main brands—Sweet'n Low, Splenda, and NutraSweet—is made from a different chemical combination.

Sweet'n Low (saccharin). Of these three, saccharin has the best and longest overall safety record. If you are eating out and only have access to these three sugar substitutes, use Sweet'n Low (usually in a pink packet). As natural sweeteners such as Truvia and PureVia become more readily available, though, you won't need to choose this or any chemical sweetener.

Splenda (sucralose). You'll find this in a yellow packet. The jury is still out regarding its long-term safety; overall, however, sucralose is believed to be okay for most people and is often found in sugar-free ice cream.

NutraSweet (aspartame). It's surprising that this sweetener ever received FDA approval for use. Although it is likely okay in moderation for most people, some individuals experience severe reactions to aspartame including seizures, headaches, memory loss, nausea, dizziness, confusion, depression, irritability, anxiety attacks, personality changes, heart palpitations, chest pains, skin diseases, loss of blood sugar control, and more. You may not realize aspartame is causing the reaction until you stop using it for seven to ten days and then retry it.

ADVANTAME

Approved in 2014 by the Food and Drug Administration, advantame can be used in products like baked goods, soft drinks, gum, candy, frozen desserts, puddings, jams and jellies, fruit juices, and as a tabletop sweetener and an ingredient in cooking. Advantame is 100 times sweeter than aspartame (Equal), so only a small amount is needed to achieve the same level of sweetness.

When You Can't Resist Sugar

If you feel you must have a sugary snack, eat one or two bites and savor it without guilt. Enjoy it and don't beat yourself up. That will only make you want to eat more. The problem is consuming too much sugar—occasional "cheats" are okay. Eighty percent of the pleasure comes from the first two bites—you don't need to gobble down the rest.

And the winner of best sweetener is… Stevia and erythritol (PureVia and Truvia)! These two natural sweeteners win hands down, followed by maltitol (for sugar-free chocolates). Natural sweeteners are just safer and better for you. So whenever you are planning to eat out, or are on the run, be sure and bring along several packets of your favorite natural sweetener to use.

That said, a chemical sweetener like aspartame, in say a diet soda, is still better than sugar, if you are trying to heal your sugar addiction. So, if your choice is between a regular soda and a diet soda with NutraSweet, and there is no other sweetener option (and water just won't do it for you at that time), enjoy the diet soda.

A key point is to use any sweetener in moderation.

OTHER HEALTHY HABITS TO HELP KICK THE SUGAR HABIT AND CURB CRAVINGS

Okay, now that you're on the path to being sugar free, it's time to think about making healthy lifestyle choices: cutting back on caffeine, adding whole foods to your diet, improving your sleep hygiene, taking a multivitamin, and drinking more pure water. Together, these new habits can make a tremendous difference in dealing with cravings, changing the way you feel, giving you energy, and in the ability to "meet life" effectively.

Cut Out Excess Caffeine

Excess caffeine aggravates the symptoms of sugar addiction. It also makes you tired, and that makes you reach for sugar to artificially boost your energy. Research shows that coffee does offer health benefits when used in moderation. (See sidebar.) Keeping this in mind, limit yourself to one to two cups of regular coffee a day and then switch to tea (preferably caffeine-free after the first cup). Use tea leaves or teabags instead of powders or bottled teas, which are high in sugar (more like soda).

If you are currently drinking more than four cups of coffee a day, cut the amount in half each week or two (as is comfortable) until you get down to one cup a day. This decreases the risk of caffeine-withdrawal headaches.

Choose Whole Foods That Won't Fuel Your Sugar Cravings

The next step is to add healthy foods to your diet that will help keep you off the sugar roller coaster. The best way to do this is to choose whole foods (i.e., unprocessed fruit, vegetables, grains, or meat). Most of these foods are also low on the glycemic index, so they won't fuel your sugar cravings.

The Many Benefits of Coffee in Moderation

Recent research has shown that a cup of Joe offers more than a way to get you through the day. It is high in helpful antioxidants that scavenge unstable molecules (free radicals) to prevent damage to the cells in the body and inhibit inflammation and, consequently, development of cardiovascular disease and high blood pressure. The *Nurses' Health Study II* showed that moderate consumption of both caffeinated and decaffeinated coffee may also lower the risk of type 2 diabetes in middle-aged and younger women. Coffee can also boost brain power, helping to preserve cognitive skills, thinking, memory, and comprehension.

The glycemic index (GI) tells you which foods raise your blood glucose fastest and highest. This is especially important for sugar addicts to keep in mind. Pure glucose gets a GI score of 100—all other foods are measured in relation to glucose. A food with a glycemic index over 85 raises blood sugar rapidly, but a food with a glycemic index under 30 does not raise blood sugar much at all. You also need to take portion size into account, of course. The term *glycemic load* combines these factors.

You'll find a glycemic index list in appendix B, which will guide you in making healthy food choices. Selecting foods with glycemic index scores that are right for you will depend both on your sugar addiction type and on how much protein, fiber, and other healthy nutrients (like vitamins and minerals) the foods contain. (We'll offer recommendations in the following chapters that discuss individual treatments.) Remember, the best approach is to listen to your body. Which foods and combinations leave you feeling the best overall?

Get Enough Sleep to Slash Sugar Cravings

It's important to sleep seven to nine hours per night. Adequate sleep optimizes energy, decreases your appetite, and slashes sugar cravings. You'll find commonsense recommendations listed below. We'll also talk more about this in chapter 6.

- Go to bed and wake up at the same time each day. This will set your internal clock (circadian day/night rhythm) to a healthy pattern. Your body loves routine.

- Don't drink alcohol right before bedtime.

- Cut off your caffeine intake at 2:00 p.m. It's okay to have a cup or two of tea or coffee in the morning, but switch to decaf after 2:00 p.m.

- If you frequently wake up to urinate during the night, do not drink a lot of fluids near bedtime.

- Keep the bedroom cool, around 65°F (18.3°C).

- Don't exercise within an hour of bedtime.

- Put the bedroom clock out of arm's reach and facing away from you so you can't see it. Looking at the clock frequently aggravates sleep problems and is frustrating.

Supplements That Help Curb Cravings

These herbs and supplements can help keep your sweet tooth under control.

Note: It's best to use all of these remedies under the guidance of your holistic health care practitioner. As with any herbal supplement, do NOT take with the medication Coumadin unless OK'd by your physician.

These next two supplements help in two main ways. They support adrenal function and decrease low blood sugar.

Ginseng. Both American and Asian ginseng can help if you crave sweets when you are under stress and are especially helpful for type 2 sugar addiction, helping to curb emotional overeating and keep blood sugar levels stable. The National Center for Complementary and Alternative Medicine (NCCAM) notes that some studies have shown that Asian ginseng may lower blood glucose, while other studies indicate possible beneficial effects on immune function. Asian (Panax) ginseng is preferred, unless you have high blood pressure, in which case choose American Ginseng. Take: 100 mg two times day.

Chromium. This herb helps keep blood sugar levels stable, thus decreasing both irritability and sugar cravings. Chromium is critical for insulin function and has been shown to be helpful in atypical (irritable) depression as well. Dose: 200 mcg per day in a good multivitamin.

The following four supplements also help in two main ways. They help with insulin resistance and lowering elevated blood sugar in diabetes. That's because, although the blood sugar is high, the sugar just cannot get into the cells. This leaves them essentially sugar starved (no matter how much sugar you eat) and leaves you craving sweets:

Berberine. This herb comes from Goldenseal and is also helpful in diabetes and for treating gut Candida and other infections. Dose: 250 mg three times day and can be as high as 500 mg three times day if it does not cause upset stomach.

Cinnamon. This has a modest effect on blood sugar, but added to foods like cereals and coffee, it adds flavor in a way that decreases the need for adding sugar.

Vitamin D. Research shows that when Vitamin D levels are low in the body, the hormone that helps turn off your appetite doesn't function and you feel hungry, no matter how much you eat. In 2009, researchers at the University of Minnesota found that those who have enough Vitamin D tend to lose more weight than those with low levels. Low Vitamin D is also associated with increased diabetes risk. Take: 400 to 2000 IU daily as part of a good multivitamin.

Omega-3 fatty acids. Found in cold water fish like cod and salmon, omega-3 fatty acids are good for healthy brain function and mood, but are also good for glucose control. In a study conducted by researchers from the University of South Australia and published in the medical journal *Public Health Nutrition* (2013), a higher intake of omega-3 fatty acids can help reduce insulin resistance, in turn lowering the risk of type 2 diabetes. Eat two to three servings of oily fish (such as salmon or tuna) a week or supplement your intake of omega-3 fatty acids with Vectomega (by EuroPharma). Just take one Vectomega each day, which replaces eight to ten fish oil caps!

Supplement with a Good Vitamin Powder to Stop Sugar Cravings

Getting optimal nutritional support is important for overall health in general. Every sugar addict can benefit from a good powdered multivitamin. That's because inadequate levels of nutrients will trigger food cravings in general and sugar cravings in particular, as your body instinctually seeks to get the nutrition it needs.

Because human beings need more than fifty key nutrients, you'll find that using vitamin powders makes sense. One drink can replace at least thirty-five tablets of supplements. In appendix A, you'll find the vitamin powder we recommend. Check off treatment #1.

Drink Water to Aid Sugar Detoxing

You will have a tougher time kicking sugar if you don't stay hydrated. Water helps the machinery of the body function and lets the body rid itself of toxins. How much water should you drink a day? Check your mouth and lips every so often. If they are dry, you are thirsty and need to drink more water. It's that simple.

But drinking tap water isn't the way to go. Tap water's great for cleaning dishes and clothes, but not so good for human consumption. Tap water just isn't pure and can be full of organisms and contaminants. Bottled water has problems, too. Many brands of bottled water are simply tap water, and cost has little to do with quality. As the joke goes, Evian spelled backward is "naïve." But we need to have easy access to healthy water. So how can you tell what is best?

When drinking bottled water, use water that is purified by reverse osmosis and carbon block filtration. For home use, a good water filter is best.

IT'S TIME TO TREAT YOUR INDIVIDUAL SUGAR ADDICTION

Now that you've learned all about the healing practices that can help each and every sugar addict, it's time to get down to specifics. In the following four chapters, you'll find specific treatment plans for each addiction type.

As we mentioned before, you may fit more than one type. If that's the case, start with the first one that applies to you and then move on to the next one. As you go through each chapter that applies to your type, mark down in appendix A the treatments you'll be using. By the time you've finished part II, you'll have a program that will enable you to break your addiction and improve your overall health—so you can feel great!

Switching from Sugary Drinks to Healthy Water

Water is the best thirst quencher and contains no sugar or calories. But not all water is created equal. Here are some tips:

- Avoid "enhanced water," which is little more than flavored sugar water.

- Choose bottled water that's been purified by reverse osmosis and carbon block filtration.

- Install a water filter in your home and/or workplace. When purchasing a filtration system, consider: 1) effectiveness, 2) purchase price, and 3) cost per gallon to operate. See appendix D for a good resource.

- Don't leave water in plastic bottles in a hot place (such as your car in the summertime).

- Fill a stainless steel container with filtered water and carry it with you, instead of drinking water in plastic bottles.

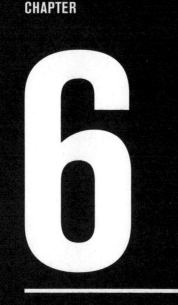

TREATMENT FOR TYPE 1 SUGAR ADDICTS: USE THE SHINE PROTOCOL TO REPAIR YOUR BODY

In order to recover from type 1 sugar addiction, you will need to take a whole-body approach to treating the fatigue that drives your addiction to sugar. This starts with eliminating "loan shark" energy drinks and sodas and modifying how much coffee you drink. If you are a type 1 sugar addict who only has mild fatigue, these next 3 steps will often be all you need to feel great:

1. Rest your body. Get eight hours of sleep a night as often as possible. Poor sleep stimulates appetite, increases sugar cravings, and contributes to weight gain.

2. Feed your body. Cut back on the junk food in your diet, stay hydrated (with water), and get simple but highly effective nutritional support.

3. Use your body. Getting exercise and sunshine will improve insulin sensitivity and help decrease sugar cravings.

If you are a type 1 sugar addict who has more severe fatigue, you may benefit from the SHINE Protocol.

THE SHINE PROTOCOL

We recommend what we call the SHINE approach to end type 1 sugar addiction. It includes predominantly natural remedies and, when needed, prescription medications. Addressing all of these factors together enables you to heal your body and feel better than ever before. SHINE stands for the following:

Sleep. Optimize sleep and treat sleep disorders.

Hormonal support. Hormones regulate your body's functioning, including energy production and sugar cravings.

Infections. Infections, including sinusitis and recurrent colds and flus, drain energy.

Nutritional support. Use vitamins, minerals, and other nutrients to heal your body and stop sugar cravings.

Exercise. Walk (or do another type of exercise) for thirty to sixty minutes a day. If possible, exercise outside so you can get sunshine as well.

R̶x̶ **YOUR WELLNESS PRESCRIPTION**

☐ 1. Get seven to nine hours of sleep per night.

☐ 2. Use natural remedies to help you sleep.

☐ 3. Don't watch the news or do things that make you feel bad, especially before bed.

SLEEP: GET A GOOD NIGHT'S SLEEP TO STOP SUGAR CRAVINGS
Why Sleep Is So Important

In the past century, the average amount of sleep a person in the United States gets per night has decreased from nine hours to around six and a half hours. This is like the body taking a 30 percent pay cut! An estimated 45 million Americans fit the official definition of chronic insomnia: having trouble falling asleep or staying asleep or waking up too early, at least three times a month, for more than a month.

The result?

Fatigue, pain, obesity, and sugar cravings. When you don't get enough sleep (between seven and nine hours a night), you end up feeling tired and craving sugar to artificially generate energy.

Poor Sleep = Sugar Cravings = Weight Gain

A lack of sleep has also been shown to directly increase appetite and weight gain. As researchers at Laval University in Quebec City, Quebec, found, if you aren't getting enough sleep, you have a 30 percent risk of becoming obese and can expect an average weight gain of five pounds (see chapter 1).

You'll gain weight if you don't sleep enough because deep sleep regulates growth hormone (the "fountain of youth hormone") and controls the production of leptin and ghrelin. Together, these three hormones regulate appetite. This means if you don't get enough sleep, you'll want to eat more, especially sugar! Growth hormone also helps turn fat into muscle. Increased muscle mass helps you burn calories more efficiently and improves insulin sensitivity—in other words, it stops sugar cravings.

Lack of sleep can lead to insulin resistance. This means you cannot get sugar out of the bloodstream and into your cells where it is needed for fuel. Because of this, your body cries out for sugar but can't burn the sugar you eat. You're left endlessly craving sugar, overweight, exhausted, and even diabetic if the insulin resistance becomes severe.

When you get seven to nine hours of sleep a night, you take a huge step toward optimizing your energy, decreasing your appetite, and slashing your sugar cravings. Getting adequate, regular sleep will also leave you feeling energized—your mind will be clearer and you'll look younger and thinner. (See sidebar.) Many people find that getting optimal sleep even makes chronic pain disappear.

New Fountain of Youth: Healthy Diet, Exercise, and Sleep

A new study from UC San Francisco is the first to show that while stress can make us age faster, it can also be counteracted by exercising and eating and sleeping well. The research published in the science journal *Molecular Psychiatry* (July 2014) revealed that the study participants who adopted these three habits had less telomere shortening than the ones who didn't maintain healthy lifestyles, even when they had the same amount of stress. Telomeres are the protective caps at the ends of chromosomes that affect how quickly cells age.

Practice Good Sleep Hygiene

These habits will help you fall asleep more quickly and sleep more soundly!

- *Hot bath.* Take a hot bath before bed.

- *Cool room.* Keep your bedroom cool.

- *Caffeine-free.* Don't consume caffeine after 4:00 p.m.

- *Alcohol early.* Don't consume alcohol near bedtime.

- *Snack to snooze.* Eat a 1 to 2 ounce (28 to 55 g) high-protein snack before bedtime; otherwise, hypoglycemia (low blood sugar) will cause insomnia. Choose: a hard-boiled egg, nuts, cheese, or turkey.

- *Bedroom, not office.* Don't use your bedroom for problem-solving or work.

- *Leave the laptop out of the bedroom too.* The brightness of the computer screen can reset your body clock, wake you up, and make it more difficult to go to sleep.

- *Ignore the clock.* Put the bedroom clock out of arm's reach and facing away from you so you can't see it. Looking at the clock frequently aggravates sleep problems—and it's frustrating!

- *Solve snoring.* If your partner snores, sleep in a separate bedroom. Or get a good pair of wax earplugs that mold to the shape of the ear and use them.

- *Better bladder control.* If you frequently wake up to urinate, don't drink a lot of fluids near bedtime.

- *Exercise early.* Work out at least five or six hours *before* bedtime. (See sidebar page 162.)

Herbal Remedies for Insomnia

Okay, so you've tried the basic recommendations and still find yourself tossing and turning. It's time to take the next step, using natural remedies to help you sleep better and more soundly. More than 1.6 million U.S. adults are estimated to use complementary and alternative therapies to treat insomnia or troubled sleeping, according to a new national survey published in the *Archives of Internal Medicine.* Natural sleep aids can be safely taken long term, either as needed or every night.

Theanine: This amino acid that comes from green tea improves sleep at night and alertness during the day. That's because L-theanine aids in the formation of gamma-aminobutyric acid (GABA), which helps you sleep better. Use only brands containing the SunTheanine form (pure L-theanine). Recommended dose: 50 to 200 mg at bedtime.

Lemon balm: Like lavender, this member of the mint family is a natural relaxant. Placebo-controlled research published in the medical journal *Fitoterapia* in 1999 showed that taking 80 to 160 mg of lemon balm with 180 to 360 mg of valerian at night improved the quality of deep sleep.

Wild lettuce: The bitter cousin to ordinary garden lettuce, this herb aids insomnia and anxiety. Ancient Egyptians used a form of wild lettuce as an aphrodisiac. Research shows that it is useful as a mild sedative and even a cough suppressant. It may also decrease the symptoms of restless leg syndrome. Recommended dose: 30 to 120 mg of the extract at bedtime.

Try Flower Essences for Insomnia

Bach Flower Remedies are made from a "sun tea" of specific wildflowers or trees known for their healing properties and to help balance emotions. Take the remedy under the tongue or add a few drops to a glass of water and sip it. The Bach remedy White Chestnut helps to calm the mind and turn off repetitive thoughts that can keep you awake, while Vervain flower essence works for high-energy, high-strung people who have difficulty slowing down for sleep. For more information, visit www.bachflower.com.

Valerian: This is the go-to remedy for insomnia, and a number of studies confirm its usefulness, showing it improves deep sleep, lessens the time it takes to fall asleep, and enhances the quality of sleep, all without becoming habit forming. A review of studies in the *American Journal of Medicine* in 2006 confirms that valerian improves sleep quality safely. (Note that 5 to 10 percent of the population actually gets energized from valerian. If this happens to you, use it during the day for anxiety, but not at night for sleep.) According to the German Commission E, the expert panel that evaluates herbal medicines for the German Counterpart of the FDA, no side effects have been documented for valerian. Recommended dose: 200 to 800 mg of the extract at bedtime.

Hops: This is a native British plant (related to stinging nettles) and a member of the hemp family; the ripened cones of the female plants are used to make beer. Hops is a good herb for insomnia, muscle tension, and anxiety. A study published in *Sleep* in 2005 showed hops improves the quality of sleep without side effects. Recommended dose: 30 to 120 mg of a hops extract at bedtime.

Passionflower: A favorite herb in South America for its calming properties, passionflower is approved by the German Commission E for insomnia and nervousness. It can also be used to treat anxiety, muscle spasms, and menstrual pain. Recommended dose: 90 to 360 mg of the extract at bedtime.

Note: These six herbs can be taken separately, or they can be found in combination in the **Revitalizing Sleep Formula** (Enzymatic Therapy). See appendix A.

If you have insomnia, check off treatment #3 in appendix A. For most of you with mild to moderate insomnia, this is all you will need to sleep like a baby. If your insomnia is more severe, you can add the treatments below as needed to find a combination that lets you get your seven to nine hours of sleep a night.

Lavender: A member of the mint family, lavender is an excellent aromatherapy for sleep and relaxation. (See aromatherapy sidebar page 60.) The lavender aroma comes from the oil in the blue-purple flowers. Human clinical studies, including one by Dr. Ikue Kotsubaki and his colleagues in a hospital intensive care unit, published in the *Medical Journal of Hiroshima Prefectural Hospital* in 1999, confirm its calming, soothing, and sedative benefits. Lavender oil is now available by capsule as Calm Aid (Nature's Way) and is very helpful for both anxiety and sleep.

Use Aromatherapy for a Good Night's Sleep

Lavender is one of the best essential oils for insomnia, and it also relieves tension and anxiety. Two hours before bedtime, try taking an Epsom salt bath and before you get in, add 8 to 10 drops of lavender oil. This remedy works because Epsom salt is basically magnesium, a muscle relaxant, and lavender is a calming herb. Because the oil helps to slow nerve impulses, it can reduce irritability and bring on sleep. You can also mist your pillow with a mixture of lavender essential oil and water, put a lavender sachet under your pillow, or apply a few drops of lavender oil to your temples or neck.

Treating Sleep Disorders

You'll find lots of helpful information about these sleep disorders by visiting my website: www.endfatigue.com. If necessary, talk to your doctor about treatment. You'll find that you sleep and feel better!

- **Sleep Apnea:** The soft tissue at the back of your throat (the soft palette) obstructs the airway during sleep, repeatedly cutting off your breathing and interrupting sleep.

- **Upper Airway Resistance Syndrome:** This is a milder form of sleep apnea—difficulty breathing through the nose while sleeping.

- **Restless Legs Syndrome:** Your legs move during sleep.

- **Periodic Limb Movements in Sleep:** Your limbs move during sleep.

Use Nutritional or Other Nonprescription Supplements to Sleep Better

Many simple supplements that you can find at your health food store will help ensure a good night's sleep. These include the following:

Magnesium: Take 200 to 500 mg of magnesium at night to help you sleep better. If you get diarrhea from magnesium, use a sustained-release form. (Check off treatment #4 in appendix A.)

Calcium: Calcium can relax muscles and decrease leg cramps, thus enabling you to sleep better. For most people, though, taking calcium supplements alone instead of in combination with magnesium may cause more harm than good. It can even boost the risk of heart disease. Recommended dose: 600 mg of calcium at bedtime, along with magnesium (see above), if you have osteoporosis and need a calcium supplement.

5-Hydroxy L-tryptophan (5-HTP): 5-HTP helps produce serotonin, a neurotransmitter that makes us feel good and also helps us sleep. If you are taking medications that increase serotonin (these include antidepressants like Prozac, St. John's wort, Ultram, and Desyrel), see your holistic practitioner for correct dosing. Recommended dose: 100 to 400 mg at night.

Melatonin: This sleep-regulating hormone is made by the pineal gland and helps ensure a good night's sleep. Lower doses of 0.3 to 0.5 mg are as effective as the higher doses commonly sold. You can find Melatonin in any health food store.

How Exercise Helps Sleep and When to Do It

Making exercise a regular part of your routine has many benefits, one of which is that it improves the quality and quantity of sleep. Research at Stanford University in California showed that moderate exercise helped people get to sleep twice as fast and helped them sleep 40 minutes longer each night. But exercising too close to bedtime can keep you awake. That's because it has an energizing effect and raises your body temperature. Five or six hours later, your temperature falls, which makes sleep easier. Try exercising five or six hours before you go to bed for a minimum of twenty minutes three times a week.

Prescription Medications to Improve Sleep

If you still find you have trouble sleeping at least seven hours a night after trying the above, it is reasonable to ask your doctor to prescribe a sleep medication. Start with medications that are not addictive. A few excellent ones are as follows:

Trazodone (Desyrel): Although marketed as an antidepressant, it does not appear to be very effective for depression. It is, however, an excellent sleep aid when taken in very low doses. Recommended dose: 25 to 100 mg.

Neurontin (gabapentin): This medication is also available as a low-cost generic. It is especially helpful if nerve pain, pelvic pain, or restless leg syndrome is interfering with your sleep. Recommended dose: 100 to 400 mg at bedtime.

Flexeril: This muscle relaxant is also available as a low-cost generic. One-half to one tablet at bedtime can be very effective and will also help relieve muscle aches at night. Recommended dose: 2½ to 5 mg.

Ambien (zolpidem): A major plus of this medication is that it is short-acting, which means it leaves your body after six hours, reducing that sleep hangover you get from some medications. Recommended dose: 5 to 10 mg at bedtime. If you find you wake up during the night, it's okay to take an extra one-half to one tablet, but it is best to take no more than 10 mg total per night (it can be addictive). You can also ask your doctor to prescribe Ambien CR, which is a sustained-release formula. Recommended dose: 6.25 to 12.5 mg at bedtime.

HORMONES: HYPOTHYROIDISM CAN MAKE YOU CRAVE SUGAR

You may crave sugar because you feel tired. This can be the result of an underactive thyroid. Unfortunately, many physicians still do not realize that the majority of people who need thyroid hormone have normal blood tests. Many conventional doctors also prescribe a synthetic thyroid hormone that does not contain any active T3 thyroid hormone. It may help some people, but it is often ineffective if what you need is the T3 hormone.

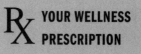

℞ YOUR WELLNESS PRESCRIPTION

If you are tired and experience weight gain, cold intolerance, or other symptoms of an underactive thyroid, you deserve a therapeutic trial of prescription natural Thyroid—even if your blood tests are normal. Try it for a few months to see whether your symptoms improve.

Because thyroid testing is unreliable and standard treatments aren't very effective, how do you get the help you need? Find a physician who will prescribe according to your symptoms, that is, unexplained fatigue, weight gain, cold intolerance, and other symptoms suggestive of an underactive thyroid. A Holistic physician (see appendix C) will likely recommend a natural form of thyroid hormone, which contains a mix of two thyroid hormones called T3 and T4. In part III, we'll talk more about treating hypothyroidism, including the importance of iron and selenium supplementation.

INFECTIONS: SUGAR ADDICTS ARE SUSCEPTIBLE TO INFECTIONS

When your energy levels go down because of chronic sugar use, your immune system is weakened, making it more likely that you will catch every bug, cold, or flu virus that goes around. Type 1 sugar addicts may be particularly vulnerable because the sugar in one can of soda is enough to suppress your body's defense forces by 30 percent for a three-hour period! This makes it critical to prevent infections that drain your energy.
Try these supplements:

Zinc: One of the most important nutrients for maintaining strong immune function, zinc can be found in high-protein foods. This is another benefit of the high-protein/low-carbohydrate diet that works best for healing sugar addicts. A good multivitamin usually contains 15 to 25mg of zinc.

Rx YOUR WELLNESS PRESCRIPTION

- [ ] 1. Take 15 to 25 mg of zinc per day.
- [ ] 2. Take 500 to 100 mg of vitamin C per day.
- [ ] 3. Stay hydrated.
- [ ] 4. Get proper rest.
- [ ] 5. Wash your hands frequently during flu season or when infections are going around.

Vitamin C: Taking vitamin C actually does make you less likely to catch a cold. This is especially true for people who are undergoing high levels of stress. A review of the medical literature published in the *Journal of Military Medicine* in 2004 showed that in five studies participants in the vitamin C group experienced a 45 to 91 percent reduction in common cold incidence. Three other trials found an 80 to 100 percent reduction in the incidence of pneumonia in the vitamin C group.

It is hard to get more than 60 to 100 mg a day from your diet, and many food sources high in vitamin C (like fruit juices) are also high in sugar, making them more problematic than helpful. For most people, 500 mg a day of vitamin C in a good multivitamin is plenty for prevention. During an infection, taking higher doses can help you recover more quickly.

Stay hydrated: Your body's first line of defense against most respiratory infections (such as colds and flu) is the moist surface linings in your nose, mouth, throat, and lungs called mucosal linings. Your body generates special "troops" (called IgA antibodies) that work best in moist environments. When you're dehydrated and these surfaces are dry, you are disarming your troops. The solution? Occasionally check your mouth and lips. If they are dry, so are the rest of the mucosal linings in your respiratory system. Drink some water.

Get proper rest: We've discussed sleep already, but it's worth revisiting here. You may have noticed that during an infection, a fever increases while you are sleeping (this is especially noticeable in children). This is because much of your defense operation occurs at night, during sleep. Research by Professor Carol Everson at the University of Tennessee has shown that a very effective way to severely suppress the immune system in an animal is to deprive it of sleep. People are no different.

Wash your hands: When a flu or other bug is going around, wash your hands often. Although being in a crowded space with someone who's hacking and sneezing feels worrisome, you are much more likely to catch a bug that has found its way onto a surface that someone else with the infection has touched. The virus then catches a ride from your hands to your mouth or nose. By simply washing your hands regularly, you'll wash these hitchhikers right down the drain.

NUTRITION: SHIFT FROM JUNK FOOD TO WHOLE FOOD

To recover from type 1 sugar addiction, you need to eliminate so-called "energy drinks," sodas, and other sugar-containing drinks from your diet. These beverages are often crammed with almost 1 teaspoon of sugar per ounce (28 ml), and the impact on your health is enormous. "One of the easiest ways to cut back on added sugars is to curtail your consumption of sweetened beverages like soft drinks, sweet tea, alcoholic mixers, and juice drinks," agrees Kathleen Zelman, MPH, RD, LD, WebMD's director of nutrition. Instead, drink diet sodas that contain stevia, Truvia, or PureVia and substitute stevia, PureVia, or Truvia for sugar in your tea, coffee, and other beverages.

You also have to eat right. That's because not having enough vitamins, minerals, and other nutrients causes fatigue, which leads to sugar cravings as your body tries to get the nutrients it needs. The short-lived energy boost you get from the sugar is physically costly.

Does Drinking Alcohol Make You Crave Sugar?

Alcohol is not a problem for most people when used in moderation and can even provide health benefits. Red wine, for example, contains compounds called resveratrol that help to lower "bad" cholesterol and improve heart health. However, there is a cross addiction between sugar and alcohol. This is one reason why alcoholics often crave sugar. If you find drinking makes you crave sugar, it's smart to stop or cut back. If alcohol is causing other problems and you want to quit, check out Alcoholics Anonymous, a 12 step program that has helped many people stop drinking. For more information, visit www.aa.org.

℞ YOUR WELLNESS PRESCRIPTION

☐ 1. Eliminate so-called "energy drinks" loaded with sugar and caffeine.

☐ 2. Eliminate excess sugar.

☐ 3. Limit caffeine intake.

☐ 4. Eat whole foods instead of processed ones.

☐ 5. Drink good-quality water.

☐ 6. Increase salt intake if you have low blood pressure.

☐ 7. Get nutritional support with a good vitamin powder.

☐ 8. Turbocharge your energy with ribose.

☐ 9. Optimize nutrients, particularly B vitamins.

The closer you get to a whole foods diet, the healthier you'll be. "Whole food" means the way fruits, vegetables, grains, and meat were before they got processed. Over time, you will find that you actually prefer eating this way because it tastes better. You're not denying yourself pleasure. You are simply learning better ways to enjoy your food and make healthy eating a habit over the long term.

Type 1 sugar addicts can benefit most from choosing to eat low-glycemic index (GI) foods that won't fuel your sugar cravings. You'll find a glycemic index in appendix B that will help you make appropriate choices.

Grains and Cereals

Although grains and cereals (more about these in a minute) have a fairly high glycemic index score, they help provide nutritional balance in your diet, so eating them in moderation, say seven servings a week, is okay for type 1 sugar addicts. Moderation means the equivalent of one to two slices of bread per day. Always choose whole-grain products instead of those made with white flour. Remember, 18 percent of the average American's calories come from white flour, which acts like sugar as it breaks down in your body.

When it comes to choosing a cereal, consider this: Recently, the Environmental Working Group (EWC) analyzed more than 1,500 cereals, including 181 for kids. They found that eating a bowl of kids' cereal each day adds up to eating 10 pounds (4.5 kg) of sugar each year! To reduce sugar consumption, the EWC recommends reading nutrition labels, buying cereals with no more than a teaspoon (equivalent to 4 grams) per serving, or preparing unsweetened hot cereals.

After a few weeks, your taste buds will adapt to the lower amount of sugar and you'll actually taste the natural sweetness of your food. Read the labels so you're sure what you're getting—some healthy-sounding granolas contain plenty of sugar or other sweeteners such as honey.

When it comes to pasta, think whole wheat, too. The glycemic index ratings for standard wheat pastas depend on thickness—the thicker the pasta, the lower the GI score—and the way it is cooked. Al dente pasta—somewhat firm and still a bit chewy—has the lowest score. The longer you cook pasta, the softer it becomes and the higher the GI ranking.

Many restaurants have whole-grain options on their menus (even Subway and Quiznos offer subs with whole-grain bread). If no whole-grain option is available, skip bread or pasta at that meal. If rice is offered, opt for brown or wild rice instead of white. Unless whole-grain pastas are an option, pass on the spaghetti at your favorite Italian restaurant and try an entrée like a chicken marsala or chicken Parmesan instead.

Whole grains are kind of like beer for some folks—they're an acquired taste. Don't make the switch all at once. Rather, do it over a period of four to twelve weeks. Soon you'll find that whole grains actually have more flavor than the pasty white stuff.

Reduce Sugar and White Flour as Painlessly as Possible

When eliminating foods with sugar and white flour from your diet, begin with those that give you the least pleasure. For example, if you are a pizza lover (and it is tricky finding whole-grain pizza at restaurants), allow yourself to occasionally have a few slices. Choose thin crust. Meanwhile, cut out other white-flour products that offer less pleasure.

Fruits and Vegetables

Fruits tend to be high in sugar and therefore rank high on the glycemic index, so it's best to just eat them in small amounts to satisfy your sugar cravings in a way that's healthy. Limit yourself to one or two servings of raw whole fruit a day. Avoid fruit juices, fruit drinks, and canned fruits, all of which contain massive amounts of sugar.

Choose vegetables with a glycemic index score of less than 55 and aim for three to five servings a day. A few vegetables, like carrots and peas, score high on the glycemic index. Others, such as potatoes, are predominantly starches and act like sugar in your body (and also rank high on the glycemic index). Most vegetables, however, can be eaten without problems and offer excellent nutritional support, providing vitamins, minerals, and fiber.

As you can see from the glycemic index list in appendix B, most nonstarchy vegetables actually fall near zero on the glycemic index, making them very healthy for sugar addicts. Raw vegetables are healthier than steamed or boiled (a lot of good stuff goes out in the cooking water). Salads are good options, although iceberg lettuce is very low in vitamins and minerals—eat mixed greens or spinach instead. Frozen vegetables are better than canned.

Although they have a higher glycemic index value, beans and legumes are high in protein, vitamins, minerals, and fiber, making them a healthy choice for sugar addicts. Enjoy up to four servings a day.

Meat, Eggs, Seafood, and Dairy

Meats, eggs, and seafood are high-protein foods that generally score zero on the glycemic index, and you can eat as much of these as you like. Eggs and some types of meat, for example, are a good choice for breakfast—skip the potatoes and toast. Make these protein foods the main dish in most of your meals, adding beans/legumes, vegetables, and greens for balance as directed in the GI reference guide.

Fish is especially healthy (unless it is fried, which often destroys the health benefits). In fact, the omega-3 oils found in fish can be more beneficial for mood and depression than prescription antidepressants, in addition to lowering the risk of heart disease. If possible, buy meat that is organic and hormone-free. The hormones, chemicals, and antibiotics added to meat and poultry can aggravate your sugar cravings.

Type 1 sugar addicts can also eat up to four servings of dairy products per day, but again, choose organic milk, cheese, and yogurt (see sidebar) whenever you can.

When eating out, organic may not be an option. That's okay. It's not necessary to eliminate all the problem foods in your diet; simply trim them back. Give yourself permission to indulge in an occasional meal that's unhealthy if you really enjoy it. As we said earlier, begin by cutting out the "bad" things that give you the least pleasure and savor the ones you truly love in moderation.

Nutritional Supplementation

Even our best efforts at eating a nutritious diet can leave us short nutritionally. In fact, it's very rare to get the optimal amount of vitamins and other nutrients from a standard Western diet today. The reason? Soils have become depleted through mass farming, which translates into less nutritious foods. Food processing also removes nutrients. Adding sugar and white flour to the diet doesn't help either, as you already know. Therefore, it's smart to supplement with a good multivitamin. But it's difficult to get optimal nutritional support in tablet form unless you take handfuls of pills.

The good news is that vitamin powders simplify the process dramatically, enabling you to get overall nutritional support in a single drink each day. Many good vitamin powders are available. You'll find more information about these and other supplements in appendix A. Check off treatment #1. In the meantime, here are the nutrients type 1 sugar addicts need for optimal health.

Dairy Foods Help Prevent Type 2 Diabetes

All saturated fats are not the same. New research shows that the saturated fat in cheese, yogurt, and other dairy products may protect against type 2 diabetes. Scientists at Cambridge University and the Medical Research Council studied the diets of more than 340,000 people to see if there was link between saturated fat and the development of diabetes. The results? Red meat, fried food, alcohol, and carbs bad, dairy products good. Keep this mind the next time you make up your shopping list.

Ribose: When you are exhausted, your body craves sugar as it tries to get an energy boost. Sugar is used by the body as fuel, where it is "burned" to recycle energy. But because sugar is used chronically and excessively, it is toxic. But a special type of sugar called ribose is an excellent nutrient for energy production. Your body treats ribose differently and preserves it for the vital work of actually making the energy molecule that powers our hearts, muscles, brains, and every other tissue in the body, in addition to its role in making DNA and RNA.

Research has repeatedly shown that ribose is the key building block to stimulate energy recovery. In fact, the main energy molecules in your body (ATP, FADH, etc.) are made of ribose plus B vitamins or phosphate.

Unlike sugar, ribose does not raise blood glucose or feed yeast overgrowth, yet it looks and tastes like sugar. Consequently, sugar addicts can use it as a sugar substitute. It actually has a negative value on the glycemic index. Ribose even tends to lower blood sugar in diabetics and may contribute to weight loss as well.

Ribose will give you a powerful energy boost. It's also great for athletes who want to enhance their strength and stamina. Start with a 5,000 mg scoop of ribose three times a day for three to six weeks and then decrease to one scoop twice a day. If you get hyper from being too energized, lower the dose. Try it for a month and prepare to be amazed!

Any brand of ribose is okay, as long as it is made in the United States, is in powder form, and you take the proper dose. Quality control problems have occurred outside of the U.S., so your best bet is to buy a brand that uses "Bioenergy" ribose. We suggest using the Corvalen form, as this has the best quality and research behind it. Two studies at our Chronic Fatigue and Fibromyalgia Research Center, published in *The Journal of Alternative and Complementary Medicine* and *The Open Pain Journal*, showed that ribose increased energy an average of 60 percent after only three weeks. Adequate ribose cannot be found in any multivitamin, so you'll need to supplement with this nutrient separately. (You can, however, mix it into your vitamin powder). Check off treatment #2 in appendix A.

Iron: Placebo-controlled research done by Dr. Verdon and his research team and published in 2003 in the *British Medical Journal* showed that in fatigued women (who did not have anemia), taking iron supplements decreased their fatigue by 29 percent after one month. Most of the women in the study had technically normal iron levels, but their ferritin levels were lower than 50.

If you experience fatigue, ask your physician to do a blood test called a ferritin level. If it comes back under 60 (normal is anything over 12), taking iron is helpful. If it is over 60, you likely don't need iron (unless you have hair loss, in which case supplement with iron until your ferritin is over 100).

If your ferritin is above the upper limit of normal, have your doctor check you and your family members for a common hereditary disease of excess iron (called hemochromatosis). If found, it is very easy to treat. If missed, it can be fatal, and taking iron when it is too high is toxic.

B vitamins: B Vitamins and magnesium play a critical role in energy production for type 1 sugar addicts. Energy molecules are made up of B vitamins plus ribose. B vitamins are also important for immunity, nerve and brain function, and much more. You can find the necessary B vitamins in a good quality B-complex vitamin formula or the vitamin powders we recommend. Let's take a look at each of the individual B vitamins as well as magnesium to understand how they can benefit type 1 sugar addicts.

B_1, thiamine: In addition to being important for energy production, vitamin B_1 is essential for proper brain functioning—it's especially helpful to those sugar addicts who experience "brain fog." Research shows that supplementation with vitamin B_1 can even decrease the risk of developing complications of diabetes. For example, researchers at the University of Warwick who published their findings online in the journal *Diabetologia* in 2008 discovered high doses of thiamine can reverse the onset of early diabetic kidney disease. It also makes you more clearheaded, composed, and energetic. Recommended daily dose: 75 mg.

B_2, riboflavin: This B vitamin is critical for energy production. In higher doses (75 to 400 mg per day), it has been repeatedly shown to decrease the frequency of migraines (a common problem in sugar addicts) by 67 percent after six to twelve weeks, according to several placebo-controlled studies, including one published in the journal *Neurology* in 1998. Recommended daily dose: 75 mg.

B_3, niacin: Niacin is a key part of the energy molecule NADH (which also helps make the neurotransmitter dopamine). Niacin may also prevent Alzheimer's. Recommended daily dose: 50 mg.

B_6, pyridoxine: Vitamin B_6 serves many critical functions, including enhancing immune function. A common problem for type 1 sugar addicts is fluid retention, and B_6 can help this, too. Recommended daily dose: 45 mg.

B$_{12}$: Vitamin B$_{12}$ is another key nutrient involved in energy production and brain function. Recommended daily dose: 500 to 1,000 mcg.

Folic acid/folate: Supplementing with 800 mcg of folate a day can improve memory. In a study published in the medical journal *Lancet* in 2007, 818 cognitively healthy people ages fifty to seventy-five took either folic acid or a placebo for three years. On memory tests, the supplement users had scores comparable to people 5.5 years younger; on tests of cognitive speed, the folic acid helped participants perform as well as people 1.9 years younger. Recommended daily dose: 400 to 800 mcg.

Magnesium: Magnesium is critical for producing energy in your muscles. A deficiency of magnesium causes muscles to spasm and shorten, producing the achiness sometimes seen in type 1 sugar addicts. Magnesium deficiency can contribute to obesity by causing insulin resistance. In a University of Virginia study by colleagues, published in *Diabetes Care* in 2005, this association was even shown to occur in children. In addition, people with high magnesium intakes who were followed over a fifteen-year period showed a 31 percent lower chance of developing metabolic syndrome, a common form of insulin resistance flared by excess sugar intake and a major cause of heart attacks. Magnesium supplementation over time also decreases the frequency of migraine headaches, a common problem among sugar addicts. Recommended daily dose: 150 to 400 mg.

EXERCISE: BUILD ENERGY TO REDUCE SUGAR DEPENDENCY

Start slowly—take a thirty-minute walk four or five times a week. Your goal is to feel "good tired" after exercising and better the next day, not worse! Do not push yourself beyond what is comfortable—especially if you aren't accustomed to getting regular exercise. Otherwise, you're likely to crash and give up your exercise program.

Condition your body by increasing the length of time you walk by one minute each day, as you're able. When you get up to one hour a day, you can increase the intensity of your exercise. Consider including aerobics or swimming, for instance. Schedule a regular time to exercise with friends—make it a social occasion. This way, you are more likely to actually do it.

Exercise outside whenever possible, so you can get some sunshine, fresh air, and vitamin D in the process. We have been told to stay out of the sun to prevent cancer. However, this may not be altogether good advice. More than 90 percent of our vitamin D comes from sunshine. A number of studies have shown an association between vitamin D deficiency and diabetes, including a UCLA study published in the *American Journal of Clinical Nutrition* in 2004 that showed that people with vitamin D deficiency are at higher risk of both insulin resistance and metabolic syndrome—two conditions that drive sugar cravings. What you want to do is avoid sunburn, not sunshine.

Rx YOUR WELLNESS PRESCRIPTION

☐ 1. Get one-half to one hour of exercise four to five times a week.

☐ 2. Walk outside in the sunshine for at least thirty to sixty minutes a day.

☐ 3. Do something that's fun.

☐ 4. Start with something easy and increase the amount of exercise gradually.

Summary: An Action Plan for Type 1 Sugar Addicts

1. Follow the SHINE Protocol to kick your sugar addiction.

2. Take the quizzes at the beginning of chapters 2, 3, and 4 to see whether you also need to treat one of the other types of sugar addiction.

3. If you are experiencing the disabling exhaustion and pain of chronic fatigue syndrome or fibromyalgia, your sugar addiction requires a special intensive care approach to the SHINE Protocol, discussed in chapter 11.

4. Check off treatments #1, #2, #3, #4, and #4a in appendix A.

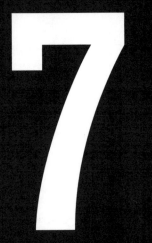

CHAPTER

7

TREATMENT FOR TYPE 2 SUGAR ADDICTS:
SUPPORT AND BALANCE YOUR ADRENAL GLANDS

Treating adrenal fatigue is essential when it comes to healing type 2 sugar addiction.
When you give the adrenal glands the nutrition they need and learn how to handle stress better,
you get off the sugar roller coaster. Supporting the adrenal glands increases their effectiveness
at producing cortisol, the primary stress hormone, which keeps your blood sugar stable.
This will help stop sugar cravings, ending the cycle of addiction.

Your treatment program includes the following steps:

1. Change your eating habits so your body can function optimally.

2. Support your adrenal "stress-handler" glands with the nutrients they need to recover.

3. Decrease the amount of unhealthy stress in your life and adopt relaxation practices such
   as deep breathing and meditation.

A DIET PLAN FOR TYPE 2 SUGAR ADDICTS

To heal the adrenal glands, it's essential that you nourish and support them through proper nutrition. Otherwise, getting well is like rolling a big boulder uphill. Bottom line? Until you examine the root causes of adrenal fatigue and your sugar addiction and change your eating habits, you won't reclaim the vital life energy you crave. It's really very simple. It just means eliminating bad eating habits and adding good ones! Let's take a look at specifics.

Cut Out Sugar, Caffeine, and White Flour

Eating the right foods is essential, so that your blood sugar remains stable. This nips sugar addiction in the bud. The first step is—you guessed it—stop eating sugar. You also need to cut back on caffeine, which worsens the symptoms of low blood sugar such as shakiness and irritability when you get hungry. Sugar and caffeine "fan the flames" of sugar addiction, hypoglycemia, and adrenal exhaustion.

It's important to also avoid processed foods that contain white flour. White flour is quickly converted into sugar in your body. Whole grains are a good alternative, but aim to decrease the amount of bread and pasta you eat overall.

To keep your blood sugar on an even keel, don't let yourself get too hungry. Eating small, frequent, high-protein, low-sugar meals (what's known as "grazing"), as opposed to the usual three large ones, can make a huge difference in the way you feel.

Rx **YOUR WELLNESS PRESCRIPTION**

☐ 1. Eliminate excessive sugars and sweets from your diet.

☐ 2. Avoid excessive caffeine.

☐ 3. Eat high-protein, low-glycemic foods.

☐ 4. Eat frequent small meals throughout the day instead of three large ones.

☐ 5. Supplement with vitamins C and B₅ (panthothenic acid), the mineral chromium, and the herb licorice to decrease the symptoms of low blood sugar.

☐ 6. Increase your salt and water intake, unless you have high blood pressure or heart failure.

Shift from Coffee to Tea to Reduce Adrenal Stress

If you need caffeine to get jumpstarted in the morning, limit yourself to one to two cups of coffee, which besides being energizing, is full of protective compounds that can help prevent many chronic diseases. After that, switch to regular tea, which usually contains less caffeine than coffee does, and even better, delicious caffeine-free herbal teas. Decaffeinated green tea is especially good because it contains theanine, which helps you stay calm and focused. Licorice tea is another good choice— it's naturally sweet and helps improve your adrenal function.

Eat High-Protein Foods to Keep Blood Sugar Stable

Meat, fish, eggs, beans, nuts, and cheese are all good sources of protein—and good foods for type 2 sugar addicts to eat. An egg is the most balanced, complete protein food you can eat. A recent review of studies by researchers from the University of Surrey published in the *Nutrition Bulletin of the British Heart Foundation* showed that eating six eggs a day for six weeks has no effect on cholesterol. Because your body breaks down protein slowly, gradually raising your blood sugar over a period of hours, eating meals and snacks that are high in protein will help you get off the sugar roller coaster.

High-protein foods also score low on the glycemic index—zero, in fact—which means you can eat as much of these as you like. Make high-protein foods the main dish in most of your meals, adding beans/legumes, vegetables, and greens for balance as directed in the GI reference guide. (See appendix B.)

Meal Recommendations for Type 2 Sugar Addicts

Breakfast: A high-protein meal at the start of the day will benefit sluggish adrenals. This means the traditional American breakfast of eggs (any style) and meat of your choice is best. Milk, yogurt, cheese, and other dairy products—up to two servings a day—are okay, too. Avoid potatoes, pancakes, and other starches. Beans, a common part of English and Mexican breakfasts, are fine. White bread is a no-no, but you can have one slice of whole-grain bread (which provides vitamins, minerals, and fiber) or a whole-grain English muffin. Limit your daily intake of whole-grain bread to no more than two servings because bread scores high on the glycemic index.

Lunch: Eat meat or fish—tuna salad, salmon, chicken, or even a hamburger on a whole wheat bun (or better yet, skip the bun altogether). Add a salad or a side vegetable (no potatoes, pasta, or high-starch vegetables) to help you feel full. Vegetables have a very low glycemic index value (choose those that rank below 55; see appendix B) and are high in vitamins, minerals, and fiber. A green salad topped with meat or fish is a good option.

Dinner: Choose high-protein foods (fish or meat) accompanied by a nonstarchy vegetable. Although beans and legumes rank higher on the glycemic index, they are also high in protein, vitamins, minerals, and fiber, making them a healthy choice for sugar addicts, particularly vegetarians. Fresh fruit can be a wonderful dessert. Eat up to one or two pieces of fresh whole fruit per day, being careful to choose ones with a glycemic index score of 42 or less.

Meeting Your Need for Protein

In an average healthy diet, 10 to 35 percent of your calories should come from protein—even 50 grams a day is enough to supply most people's nutritional needs. If you follow the guidelines presented here, you'll find it easy to meet this requirement; in fact, most of you will be getting much more than that from the diet we've recommended. The extra protein is great for type 2 sugar addicts because it supplies an energy source that will keep your blood sugar stable over many hours.

High-Protein, Low-Sugar Foods

- Meat: beef, pork, lamb, and venison

- Poultry: chicken, turkey, and game birds

- Fish and shellfish: All are okay.

- Eggs

- Nuts and seeds: All are okay.

- Dairy products: milk, plain (unsweetened) or Greek-style yogurt, cottage cheese, and hard and soft cheeses

- Vegetables: All nonstarchy vegetables are okay. Avoid or limit your consumption of potatoes, yams, beets, and related starchy vegetables to portions of 4 ounces (115g) or less, no more than four times a week. Enjoy carrots, winter squashes (e.g., acorn squash), and corn in moderation. Choose vegetables that score below 55 on the glycemic index and eat as much as you like, but aim for at least two or three servings a day.

- Beans and legumes: most beans (black, pinto, kidney, navy, etc.), lentils, split peas, tofu, and soymilk

The following list shows the amount of protein contained in some common foods:

- Hamburger patty, 4 ounces (115 g): 28 grams

- Steak, 6 ounces (170 g): 42 grams

- Most cuts of beef: 7 grams per ounce (28 g)

- Chicken breast, 3.5 ounces (100 g): 30 grams

- Fish: 6 grams per ounce (28 g)

- Tuna, 6-ounce (170 g) can: 40 grams

- Egg, large: 6 grams

- Milk, 1 cup (235 ml): 8 grams

- Cottage cheese, 1/2 cup (115 g): 15 grams

- Tofu, 1/2 cup (124 g): 20 grams

Do the math: two or three eggs at breakfast, a hamburger patty at lunch, and a chicken breast for dinner will supply plenty of protein. Snacking on nuts during the day will add even more protein.

Instead of counting grams of protein, eat what feels best to you, while simply avoiding excess sweets. As long as you are not gaining weight or getting too skinny (this diet makes it easier to lose weight), and you feel better, your eating approach is working.

Snack Smart to Stabilize Your Blood Sugar

Snacks are an important component in your meal plan because they help keep your blood sugar stable. As a general rule, type 2 sugar addicts should eat every couple of hours during the day. Enjoy a snack about two to three hours after lunch. A bedtime snack will keep your blood sugar stable while you sleep. A few ounces (85 to 115 g) of turkey is a good option at bedtime—it balances your blood sugar and contains tryptophan, which may also improve your sleep.

During the day, snack on mixed nuts and cheeses. Keep these "smart snacks" handy if your blood sugar starts to drop (i.e., if you feel irritable or shaky). Hard-boiled eggs make great snacks, too.

Nuts have an interesting side benefit. Research shows that eating 4 to 8 ounces (115 to 225 g) of walnuts lowers your cholesterol level, without causing weight gain. This seems to be the case for most nuts, perhaps because nuts are high in an essential fatty acid called alpha-linolenic acid, which seems to increase your metabolism. In 2003, the FDA announced that producers of nuts (such as peanuts, almonds, and walnuts) could make the health claim linking nut consumption to reduced heart disease risk.

Which Sweets Can You Eat?

We know giving up the sugary foods you love is a tall order, but little changes can make a big difference. For example, you can get the sugar taste you crave by using stevia and/or erythritol, two natural sweeteners, instead of sugar. These can be found in combination in Truvia and PureVia. You can also buy drinks and food products that use these natural sweeteners. Learn more about sugar substitutes in chapter 5: Healing Practices for All Sugar Addicts.

A Quick Fix to Balance Blood Sugar

When your blood sugar is dropping and you start craving sugar, it only takes a little sugar to bring your blood sugar levels back up to normal. In fact, a single Tic Tac, one packet of sugar, or half a Lifesaver will do the trick. Here's the secret: the sugar must be absorbed under your tongue, so it immediately goes into your bloodstream, literally within seconds. Follow up with a high-protein snack so your blood sugar stays steady.

Rather than reaching for cookies or donuts, eat a few squares of antioxidant-rich dark chocolate instead (skip the milk and white varieties). Savor every bite and you won't need more. Remember, moderation is key, so go for quality instead of quantity.

If you need a "sugar fix," turn to whole fruit with a low glycemic index rating. Avoid sugar-packed fruit juices and drinks. Orange juice gives you an instant sugar rush, but eat an orange and you'll feel only a slight rise in your blood sugar. This is because the fiber naturally found in whole fruit causes the small amount of sugar in the fruit to be absorbed slowly over several hours' time. An orange contains 2 to 4 teaspoons (8 to 16 g) of natural sugar that your body will absorb over a period of one to two hours, whereas 16 ounces (475 ml) of orange juice contains 12 teaspoons (48 g) of sugar that will be absorbed in twenty minutes!

This diet does *not* forbid all sweets. We simply recommend that you eat them in very small amounts. For example, if you are dining out with friends and you see a dessert to die for on the menu, share that tempting treat with a friend. Eat one or two bites and really savor the taste. Your taste buds get quickly saturated—80 percent of the pleasure comes from the first couple of bites.

Increase Your Water and Salt Intake to Improve Adrenal Function

Your adrenal glands help your body get through stressful periods by maintaining your blood sugar, blood volume, and blood pressure. Low adrenal function makes it hard to hold on to the salt and water needed to maintain a proper blood pressure, so you're likely to become dehydrated unless you drink more water and eat more salt. (Salt is kind of like a sponge that keeps water in your body.) How much water you lose during stress varies from person to person.

Sodas, fruit juices, and caffeinated beverages only exacerbate the problem. Increase your water intake according to what feels best to you. Check your mouth and lips. If they feel dry, drink up.

In addition to drinking more water, you'll need to increase your salt intake. We know, we've heard the myth that salt is bad for you. It's not. Research has repeatedly shown that higher salt intake is associated with longer life. Study after study shows that the people with the highest salt intake live the longest. This was recently reconfirmed in a study using the NHANES database, which is the most respected nutritional database in the country. As we've seen, your adrenals help you hold on to salt and water in order to maintain adequate blood pressure. In fact, when you have underactive adrenal glands, you will often experience salt cravings.

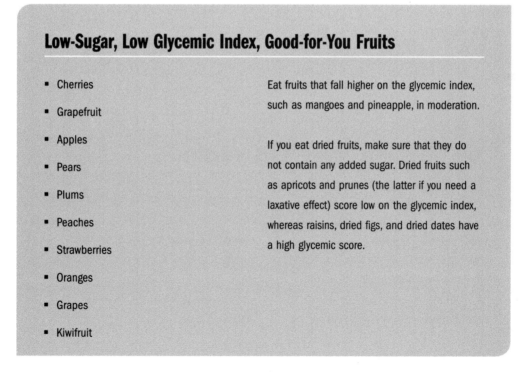

Low-Sugar, Low Glycemic Index, Good-for-You Fruits

- Cherries

- Grapefruit

- Apples

- Pears

- Plums

- Peaches

- Strawberries

- Oranges

- Grapes

- Kiwifruit

Eat fruits that fall higher on the glycemic index, such as mangoes and pineapple, in moderation.

If you eat dried fruits, make sure that they do not contain any added sugar. Dried fruits such as apricots and prunes (the latter if you need a laxative effect) score low on the glycemic index, whereas raisins, dried figs, and dried dates have a high glycemic score.

Low blood pressure or getting light-headed when you stand up could also indicate that you need more salt. If you sweat a lot, especially during the summertime, you're losing salt.

But you won't meet all of your needs with processed salt. That's because salt is meant to have many other minerals in it besides sodium and chloride. Unfortunately, normal food processing removes dozens of the minerals that are critical for life. The answer? When convenient, use natural sea salt. In addition to supporting your adrenal glands, sea salt supplies other necessary minerals such as magnesium.

Sea salt does not provide much iodine though, so using iodized salt and taking a good vitamin powder with 150 to 200 mcg of iodine (plus other necessary minerals) is also helpful. If you have high blood pressure or congestive heart failure, however, it is usually best not to increase your salt intake, unless your health practitioner approves it.

Fluid retention (puffy fingers and ankles) often paradoxically occurs even when you're dehydrated. That's because the fluid isn't staying in your blood vessels where it should be—it's leaking into your tissues. If your rings are too tight from fluid retention, it usually indicates either a need for more vitamin B_6 (up to 45 mg a day) or that you have an underactive thyroid (see more about this in chapter 15).

Take Chromium to Optimize Insulin Function

Chromium, a mineral found in tiny amounts in the human body, is especially critical for people with reactive hypoglycemia (low blood sugar during stress). Research published in the *Journal of the American College of Nutrition* in 1997 showed that taking chromium can decrease the symptoms of low blood sugar. Think of it as "taking the edge off" by optimizing insulin function. A side benefit? It may even help you lose weight. A good multivitamin will provide the necessary 200 mcg a day.

SUPPORT YOUR ADRENALS WITH SUPPLEMENTS

Supplements can help replace what your weakened adrenals are unable to supply. Taking the supplements recommended below will increase your energy, keep it stable throughout the day, and decrease episodes of low blood sugar, which drive your sugar cravings. In addition, this wellness prescription will improve your overall immune function. Once your adrenals are healed, you'll find you get sick less often.

Adrenal Extracts

To support your adrenal glands and kick sugar addiction for good, it also helps to supplement with adrenal glandulars. Taking this supplement is the quickest way to give your adrenal glands the raw materials they need to function properly. When you take them, you directly feed your adrenal glands to make them stronger. This means your adrenal glands will be able to make more of the hormone cortisol that maintains your blood sugar at proper levels. This helps keep you from crashing, relying on sweets, and continuing the cycle of addiction.

Adrenal glandulars are simply an extract of the key nutrients found in adrenal tissue taken from cows and pigs. Just as eating beef or pork (basically muscle tissue from these animals) gives you protein to build muscles, ingesting small amounts of gland tissues from these animals can support healthy gland function.

℞ YOUR WELLNESS PRESCRIPTION

☐ 1. Take 200 to 500 mg of adrenal extract daily.

☐ 2. Take 200 to 400 mg per day of a licorice extract standardized to contain 5 percent of the active agent glycyrrhizin.

☐ 3. Take 300 to 1,000 mg of vitamin C daily.

☐ 4. Take 100 to 300 mg of pantothenic acid daily.

☐ 5. Take 500 to 1,000 mg of tyrosine daily.

☐ 6. Take other glutathione (GSH) raising nutrients, including N-acetyl-cysteine, 250 to 600 mg per day; glutamine, 500 to 1,000 mg per day; and glycine, 500 to 1,000 mg per day.

☐ 7. Take a good-quality powdered vitamin-mineral supplement.

☐ 8. Discuss using the bio-identical hormones cortisol and DHEA with your holistic practitioner.

It is critical, however, that you get adrenal glandulars from a reliable source so you know that the extract contains the actual nutrients you need. Good brands include Enzymatic Therapy, ITI, and Standard Process. It is also important that purity and potency are guaranteed, and that the extracts come from cows and pigs that are not at risk of transmitting infections. Recommended daily dose: 200 to 500 mg of adrenal extract.

Take Licorice to Reduce Sugar Cravings

Licorice slows the breakdown of adrenal hormones such as cortisol, which means more of the hormones are available to stabilize blood sugar. This helps break your sugar addiction by reducing cravings. Not only does licorice supply the body with more of the critical adrenal hormones it needs, but it also helps heal the stomach and treat indigestion (it is as effective as Tagamet). Recommended daily dose: 200 to 400 mg of an extract standardized to contain 5 percent of the active agent glycyrrhizin.

Do not take higher doses of licorice if you have high blood pressure because too much licorice can cause excess adrenal function and worsen high blood pressure.

Vitamin C Helps Stabilize Blood Sugar

Your body's highest levels of vitamin C are found in the adrenal glands and brain tissues. Urinary excretion of vitamin C increases during stress because it is drawn from your body's storehouses and used. The U.S. recommended daily allowance (RDA) for vitamin C is 60 mg, which may be enough to prevent scurvy or other deficiency diseases, but is nowhere near what you need for optimal health.

Because of its role in optimizing adrenal function, vitamin C is critical for the production of the hormone cortisol, which helps keep blood sugar stable during stress. Consequently, vitamin C decreases the symptoms of low blood sugar and associated sugar cravings.

Vitamin C offers other benefits as well. Too little vitamin C in the bloodstream has been found to correlate with increased body fat and waist measurements. Research conducted at Arizona State University and published in the *Journal of the American College of Nutrition* in 2005 showed that the amount of vitamin C in the bloodstream is directly related to fat oxidation, the body's ability to use fat as a fuel source, during both exercise and at rest. Vitamin C can also boost immune function, helping to prevent the sore throats and respiratory infections that type 2 sugar addicts are predisposed to. Recommended daily dose: 300 to 1,000 mg.

Take Pantothenic Acid to Increase Cortisone Production

Although all of the B vitamins are important for good health, pantothenic acid (vitamin B_5) is critical for optimal adrenal function. Like vitamin C, pantothenic acid helps increase the production of cortisol, which keeps blood sugar stable. A lack of pantothenic acid causes shrinking of your adrenal glands. Although the daily "adequate intake" levels are set at 5 mg, optimal levels are 100 to 300 mg daily. Some physicians suggest even higher levels for adrenal support.

Tyrosine Helps Balance Your Blood Sugar

Tyrosine is the amino acid (protein building block) your body uses to make adrenaline, another adrenal stress hormone. In addition, this nutrient also makes the thyroid hormone (critical for energy) and the brain chemical neurotransmitter dopamine, which decreases cravings of all kinds, including sugar and alcohol. Dopamine also decreases depression and improves mood, so you're less likely to turn to sugar for a quick high.

Glutathione Supports Insulin Function

Glutathione, a mix of three amino acid proteins (and a critical antioxidant as well), supports insulin function, stabilizing blood sugar and helping to decrease sugar cravings. It is an important nutrient for maintaining optimal blood sugar levels. Taking glutathione supplements by mouth, though, doesn't raise glutathione levels because it's destroyed by stomach acid.

Fortunately, your body can make glutathione if you take the amino acids L-cysteine in the form of N-acetylcysteine (250 to 600 mg a day), glutamine (500 to 1,000 mg a day), and glycine (500 to 1,000 mg a day). Taking vitamin C also increases glutathione levels.

Simplify Your Nutrient Needs with Powdered Multivitamins

All of the adrenal-supporting nutrients discussed above can be obtained easily by taking a good vitamin powder (which is important for all sugar addicts) and one or two capsules of a good combination adrenal support product. (Check off treatments #1 and 5 in appendix A.)

Treat Severe Adrenal Exhaustion with Bio-Identical Adrenal Hormones

For most readers, the supplements mentioned above will be adequate to treat your adrenal exhaustion. But if you still have severe fatigue, insomnia, or very low blood pressure (under 100/70), or if you crash with minor exertion and have low blood sugar, it's time to take the next step: bio-identical adrenal hormones.

You may have heard experts discuss the pros and cons of using bio-identical hormones. Bio-identical just means that a hormone is the same as what your body normally makes. Treating underactive adrenal problems with ultra low doses of prescription bio-identical adrenal hormone, such as cortisol, and also DHEA, can ease the symptoms of low blood sugar and raise your energy—often dramatically.

The bio-identical hormones discussed below work by giving your body the hormonal support that your tired adrenal glands aren't able to provide. Meanwhile, as the adrenal glands are relieved of some of the work of making hormones, they can rest and recover. Think of bio-identicals as crutches for your tired adrenal glands. In addition to taking the burden off of the adrenals, bio-identical hormones supply adrenal hormones that help regulate key functions in the body. You can expect to see results and feel better within days.

Cortisol Helps Maintain Blood Sugar during Stress

Although taking bio-identical cortisol, which your body needs to maintain your blood sugar during stress, can be very helpful, it's best to use this treatment under the care of a holistic practitioner. This hormone is available by prescription (hydrocortisone from compounding pharmacies, or Cortef in standard pharmacies), and up to 20 mg a day has been shown in repeated studies to be quite safe. Excellent reviews on this topic have been written by professor William Jefferies and by the renowned expert on bio-identical hormones, Dr. Kent Holtorf. A study published in the *Journal of Chronic Fatigue Syndrome* in March 2008 showed that this very low dose cortisol could safely and effectively help alleviate symptoms for people who suffer from chronic fatigue syndrome and fibromyalgia.

Unfortunately, most allopathic physicians are not familiar with the distinction between using super low doses that are normally present in the body (called physiologic dosing) and very high doses (usually synthetic prednisone in doses over 5 mg a day to suppress inflammation, which is similar to over 20 mg of Cortef). These high doses can be very toxic, and most physicians mistakenly believe that the super low doses carry the same toxicity. They do not.

Why are the lower doses safer? Normally, the adrenal glands make the equivalent of 35 to 40 mg of hydrocortisone a day. Because of this, if you are using a very low dose (e.g., 5 to 20 mg of Cortef each morning) and your body doesn't want that much, it simply makes less. Higher doses will put your adrenal glands to sleep (which is dangerous) and can lead to diabetes, high blood pressure, and thinning bones.

DHEA

When the adrenal glands are exhausted, they can't produce DHEA (dehydroepiandrosterone) effectively. Interestingly, medicine has not yet figured out exactly what DHEA does, but your adrenal glands make more of this than any other hormone. Even though we are not sure how DHEA functions, when you have optimal levels of DHEA, you feel healthier and younger and have more energy. If you have a hormonally sensitive cancer, like breast cancer or prostate cancer, don't use DHEA hormone unless your physician okays it. Recommended daily dose: for most people, an optimal dose is usually 5 to 10 mg for women and 25 to 50 mg for men. DHEA is not recommended for children under the age of eighteen.

Blood level testing of DHEA is the best way to guide dosing and will help your holistic practitioner determine the correct amount of DHEA for you to take. Are you taking DHEA on your own? If so, be cautious. Too high a dose can cause acne or darkening of facial hair. Quality control problems can exist, so be discriminating. We suggest DHEA supplements from General Nutrition Center or Enzymatic Therapy (see appendix D for more information), or have DHEA made by a compounding pharmacist.

Even though we offer guidelines here, you'll probably get the best results from working with a holistic physician. More than a thousand board-certified holistic physicians are listed at www.holisticboard.org. An accredited naturopathic doctor (ND) can also be very helpful. You'll find plenty listed at www.naturopathic.org, the website of the American Association of Naturopathic Physicians. If you also have sever fatigue, CFS, or fibromyalgia, see a Fibromyalgia specialist (www.endfatigue.com, Physical Finder).

DHEA Dosing Table

Males		Females	
If the DHEA-S blood level is: (in mcg/DL)	The recommended dose of DHEA in mg/d is:	If the DHEA-S blood level (in mcg/DL) is:	The recommended dose of DHEA in mg/d is:
0–100	50	0–30	25
101–200	40	31–80	15
201–280	25	81–110	10
281–320	10	111–114	5

Mcg/DL is a unit of measurement. In this case, it shows how many micrograms of DHEA-S (DHEA sulfate, the body's storage form of DHEA) are present per deciliter (0.1 liter) of blood.

HANDLING STRESS BETTER

Giving your body and adrenal glands the nutritional and supplement support they need is only part of the solution. It's also important to examine how you respond to and handle stress. Your adrenal glands are your body's "stress handlers." Today, many of us view life as a constant crisis, which has resulted in an epidemic of adrenal exhaustion. Much of the sugar cravings, exhaustion, and irritability that are so common these days stem from adrenal exhaustion. To get well, you'll need to break this pattern, which begins with changing your thinking. Start paying attention to the things that feel good. As Abraham Lincoln once said, "Most people are as happy as they make up their minds to be."

Do a Reality Check

When you start feeling anxious and stressed out, ask yourself, "Am I in imminent danger?" If you aren't (and almost always the answer will be "no"), simply taking a moment to realize this will turn off the "fight or flight" reaction and allow your adrenals to relax. For the long term, fifteen to thirty minutes a day of basic yoga or meditation techniques can offer profound benefits. An excellent book called *The Relaxation Response* by Dr. Herbert Benson will teach you an easy and highly effective way to begin.

Focus on the Positive

Focus on what's "right" in your life. What makes you feel good? You'll find gratitude is a powerful tool for change. By being grateful for what we have, we invite in more of the same. Start by writing a gratitude list. Every morning write down five things you are grateful for—for example, your family, your job, an upcoming trip, good weather, or even a delicious cup of coffee. As you go through the day, remember to be grateful for things, both large and small. If you feel stressed, take three deep breaths, reread your list, and relax.

Eliminate the Negative

Pay less attention to the news. Newscasts are geared to sensationalize and scare viewers, so they can get you to continue watching and the news station can sell ads. Watching the news can also make you feel powerless and overwhelmed, which adds to your stress. Media broadcasts are *not* necessarily an accurate reflection of the truth. Notice how much of what is reported focuses on war, crime, disasters, economic problems, and other doom-and-gloom scenarios, instead of the positive things that are taking place. It's okay to watch for a while in order to stay informed. But as soon as you start to feel bad when you watch the news, turn off the TV. Likewise, avoid watching shows that don't make you feel good. Instead, choose to spend more time with people whose company you enjoy. You'll find these simple steps can markedly ease the stress in your life and help your adrenal glands heal.

Choose Your Thoughts

The same principle applies to your thoughts. If they don't feel good and are not helping you solve a problem, stop and change your mental "channel" to something more enjoyable. Instead of allowing your thoughts to run rampant, discipline them. Keep a few thoughts handy that always make you feel good—your children, your pet, or a hobby you love, for instance—and "switch" to them when you find yourself worrying.

After a while, the switching process will become second nature to you. You may be pleasantly surprised to discover that the concerns you found stressful fade away as you choose to focus on what feels good. Interestingly, when we choose to focus only on the things we like in people, their good qualities become magnified while their annoying traits seem to disappear (or they do) after several months of practicing this technique.

1. – Do a reality check.

2. – Focus on the positive.

3. – Let go of the negative.

4. – Choose your thoughts.

5. – Integrate relaxation practices into your day.

Bottom line? Choose to keep your attention on what feels good.

Breathe Easy

Most of us are shallow breathers—on average we only use 60 percent of our lung capacity, making us stressed and anxious. Energy breathing from the ancient Chinese practice of Qigong helps to oxygenate the blood, tissues, muscles, and organs, enhance mental focus, and reduce stress. Here's how to do it:

1. Sit or lie down in a comfortable position. Smile to relax your mind and body.

2. Place the tip of your tongue gently against the roof of your mouth and breathe through your nose in slow, gentle, deep breaths. Imagine you are using your entire body to breathe. Feel the air flowing into every part of your body.

3. As you breathe out, visualize any tiredness or stress, pain or sickness, and any doubt or worries changing into smoke. Do this for as long as you like.

4. To end your energy breathing session, take one final, slow, gentle, deep breath. Slowly open your eyes. For more information, visit www.springforestqigong.com.

Slow Down Your Thoughts with Meditation

All day long our mind is chattering with judgments and comments about what is going on around us. When you slow down and meditate, you are able, maybe for the first time, to listen to yourself and your own inner wisdom. Practicing meditation also improves blood pressure, bolsters the immune system, boosts brain power, promotes a sense of well-being, and reduces stress and anxiety. Use these three steps to begin your journey into meditation:

1. Sit in a comfortable position and close your eyes.

2. Allow your breath to fall into a natural rhythm.

3. Settle your gentle attention on your breath for 21/2 minutes or longer. When you are finished, slowly open your eyes and gently re-enter your day.

You'll find many more relaxation practices to help you handle stress in Chrystle's new book with herbalist Brigitte Mars: *The Home Reference to Holistic Health & Healing: Easy-to-Use Natural Remedies, Herbs, Flower Essences, Essential Oils, Supplements, and Therapeutic Practices for Health, Happiness, and Well-Being* (Fair Winds Press, 2015).

Summary: An Action Plan for Type 2 Sugar Addicts

1. _____ Eat a high-protein, low-sugar, low-carbohydrate diet.

2. _____ Eat frequent small meals during the day to get you off the sugar roller coaster.

3. _____ If you have low blood pressure, increase your salt and water intake.

4. _____ Support and heal your adrenal glands with supplemental nutrients.

5. _____ Take a mind-body-spirit approach to heal the adrenal glands. Choose to keep your attention on things that feel good.

6. _____ Check off treatments #1 and #5 in appendix A.

7. _____ See a holistic practitioner if symptoms persist.

8

TREATMENT FOR TYPE 3 SUGAR ADDICTS:
KILL SUGAR-CRAVING CANDIDA

Treating yeast overgrowth is essential to healing type 3 sugar addiction. When you eat too much sugar, yeast gets the upper hand, suppressing your immune system and increasing the chances of "leaky gut." When your gut walls are not intact, undigested protein gets into the bloodstream. Your immune system goes into high alert, fighting incompletely digested food, which it mistakes as "invaders." Once yeast overgrows in your gut, it can produce a chain reaction of problems, including intense sugar cravings, fatigue and moodiness, chronic sinusitis, spastic colon, allergies, and even chronic fatigue syndrome and fibromyalgia. It's a high price to pay for satisfying that sweet tooth. The good news is, you can feel good, heal your body, and still enjoy foods you love.

To beat your sugar addiction, you'll need to take a whole body approach to treating yeast overgrowth, as explained in this chapter. (In part III, you'll learn specifics about dealing with spastic colon and chronic sinusitis.)

Your treatment program includes the following steps:

1. Adopt a healthy diet that contains high-protein foods, whole grains, vegetables, and fruits that score low on the glycemic index.
2. Eliminate sugars and sweets, except for dark chocolate in moderation.
3. Use natural remedies and prescription medications to stop yeast overgrowth and keep it in check.
4. Support your immune system with natural supplements.
5. Test for and eliminate food allergies using NAET and the Elimination Diet.

A DIET PLAN FOR TYPE 3 SUGAR ADDICTS

Yeast grow by fermenting (eating) the sugar you ingest. Because of this, the most important thing is to starve them by staying away from sugar. Otherwise, you are just encouraging yeast overgrowth. Yeast use sugar to multiply, increasing your sugar cravings, suppressing your immune function, and making you feel unwell. To escape the sugar trap, focus on eating foods that are low on the glycemic index, such as protein, vegetables, and whole grains, while eliminating sugar in its many forms. (You'll find a glycemic index chart in appendix B.)

It's important to note that your symptoms of yeast overgrowth may flare up when you begin the treatment described in this chapter. When mass quantities of yeast are suddenly killed off (called a die-off or Herxheimer reaction, which can happen when treating any chronic infection), you can feel like you are coming down with the flu. To decrease the risk of this reaction, start your treatment with

R̃ YOUR WELLNESS PRESCRIPTION

☐ 1. Eliminate sugars and sweets, except for dark chocolate in moderation; better yet, eat sugar-free chocolate.

☐ 2. Use sugar substitutes, especially stevia and/or erythritol (PureVia or Truvia).

☐ 3. If you need a sugar fix, you can eat up to one or two pieces of fruit a day with a glycemic index rating of 42 or less (but don't drink fruit juices).

a sugar-free diet. Then add acidophilus (probiotics) for three weeks and anti-yeast herbals for one month before beginning the very powerful prescription antifungal medication Diflucan (fluconazole).

Supplement with a Powdered Multivitamin

Even though you may be eating healthfully, everyone can benefit from a little extra help. Food just isn't as nutritious as it was before factory farming depleted the soil. As a result, the nutrients we need may not be present in our food. Food processing also removes nutrients. Because of this, it's smart to supplement. But instead of taking a handful of pills, consider adding a good vitamin powder to your daily regimen. In most cases, this will give you everything you need. Check off treatment #1 in appendix A.

ELIMINATE SUGAR

We know giving up the sugary foods you love is a tall order. Luckily, you have choices. You can satisfy that sweet tooth with the natural sweeteners stevia and/or erythritol (the two are combined in the products PureVia and Truvia). Despite misinformation you may have heard from the makers of chemical sweeteners, stevia and erythritol are safe and natural. Add them to tea, coffee, cereal, or anywhere you'd ordinarily use sugar. You can even buy diet soda sweetened with Truvia.

If you buy pure stevia, look for a brand that is filtered; otherwise, it can taste bitter—exactly what you don't want. Two good brands are Body Ecology and Stevita. Truvia and PureVia taste good too and are rapidly becoming the best readily available choices. You'll find out more about sugar substitutes in chapter 5: Healing Practices for Every Sugar Addict.

Rather than reaching for cookies or one of the popular candy bars, eat a few pieces of antioxidant-rich dark chocolate instead (avoid milk and white varieties). Savor every bite and you won't need much. Remember, moderation is your mantra, so go for quality instead of quantity. Better yet, enjoy sugar-free chocolate. Look for brands that use a natural sugar alcohol called maltitol that the yeast cannot eat and that won't worsen your blood sugar levels.

This way of eating does *not* mean you can never have any sweets. Just eat them in very small amounts—too much and the yeast win.

If you need a "sugar fix," eat up to one or two servings daily of whole fruit with a glycemic index value less than 42. Cherries, grapefruit, apples, pears, plums, peaches, oranges, grapes, kiwifruit, and strawberries are good choices. Higher glycemic fruits such as mangoes, apricots, and pineapple are okay in moderation. Avoid sugar-packed fruit juices and fruit drinks. You may wonder, though, whether it's okay to eat "healthy" sugars, like organic honey or maple syrup. The answer is no. Avoid concentrated sugars, including honey, maple sugar, brown sugar, dried fruits, processed sugar, high-fructose corn syrup, corn syrup, jellies, pastry, cakes, and candy. Stay away from soda, too—a 12-ounce (355 ml) serving can contain 10 to 12 teaspoons (40 to 48 g) of sugar!

NATURAL REMEDIES TO TREAT YEAST OVERGROWTH

In a perfect world, yeast live in balance in the digestive system with over 500 different types of bacteria. Some bacteria is great for you, while some of it is harmful. When you take antibiotics frequently, for example, this balance is thrown off and the yeast begin to overgrow and take control.

The good news is that a mix of natural remedies plus medication is an effective way to put yeast back in their place. Natural remedies are gentler and work synergistically with the body's processes, enabling you to heal faster and feel better. These cures range from herbs that combat yeast overgrowth by acting as natural antifungals to "friendly bacteria" and yogurt, which improve the health of the gut.

Kill Yeast with Antifungal Herbs

Many natural herbs and products can kill yeast, but taking enough of any single item to be effective usually causes severe acid reflux and indigestion. Because of this, you'll want to take a low dose of several natural antifungals. Here are some effective anti-yeast herbs and their recommended doses. Check off treatment #6 in appendix A.

- Coconut oil powder (50 percent caprylic acid), 240 mg

- Oregano powder extract, 200 mg

- Uva-ursi extract, 120 mg

- Grapefruit seed extract, 160 mg

- Berberine sulfate, 200/500 mg 3 x a day

- Olive leaf extract, 200 mg

Take Probiotics to Restore Friendly Bacteria

Chronic yeast overgrowth in the gut takes months to eliminate, and it is important to replace the yeast with healthy bacteria or the yeast will simply grow back. We have more bacteria in our colons (one to ten trillion) than we do cells in our bodies. Healthy bacteria play a vital role—they help digest food, supply key nutrients, and keep unhealthy yeast, bacteria, and parasites out of your body. Restoring healthy levels of beneficial bacteria takes time (about five months) but is well worth it.

Probiotics, or "friendly bacteria" like acidophilus or milk bacteria, can help restore the balance of good bacteria in your gut. Acidophilus is found in yogurt with live and active yogurt cultures. Eating just one cup (230 g) of yogurt a day can reduce the frequency of recurrent vaginal yeast infections.

What the Research Says about Probiotics

Since the mid-1990s, interest in probiotics has grown, and more and more research is being done about their benefits. In 2008, the medical journal *Clinical Infectious Diseases* published a special issue on probiotics, which showed among other things that probiotics help treat acute diarrhea and antibiotic associated diarrhea, childhood infections, tooth decay, nasal bacteria, inflammatory bowel disease, and side effects of treatment for stomach ulcers. According to the Mayo Clinic (www.mayoclinic.org), probiotic bacteria also do the following:

- Prevent and treat vaginal yeast infections and urinary tract infections

- Treat irritable bowel syndrome

- Reduce bladder cancer recurrence

- Speed treatment of certain intestinal infections

- Prevent and treat eczema in children

- Prevent or reduce the severity of colds and flu

It is not yet clear whether the lactose (milk sugar) found in dairy products stimulate yeast growth. Lactose is less of a problem than other sugars, but until this is clarified, it is reasonable for type 3 sugar addicts to limit consumption of dairy products to three or four servings a day.

R̲x̲ YOUR WELLNESS PRESCRIPTION

☐ 1. Take anti-yeast herbs and supplements.

☐ 2. Take one Pearls Elite daily for five months to restore healthy bacteria to the colon.

☐ 3. Eat sugar-free yogurt with live bacterial cultures.

For more information about probiotics, check out the documentary, narrated by Leonard Nimoy, on DVD: *Microwarriors: The Power of Probiotics*. For more information, visit www.microwarriorsmovie.com.

Supplementing with Probiotics

You can also take acidophilus that contains good bacteria like (*Lactobacillus* and *Bifidobacterium* as a supplement, but choose a brand wisely to be sure you're getting the power of probiotics you need. Many brands don't contain enough of the "good bacteria" to rid the gut of yeast overgrowth or have dead bacteria that won't put up a fight against the yeast.

The best probiotics are made with a pearl coating so they pass through the stomach's acid environment and into the bowel intact—that's where the coating dissolves and the good bacteria in probiotics are released so they can go to work to battle yeast. Otherwise, 99.9 percent of the good bacteria are killed by stomach acid before they can do their job. Although the package claims 1 billion bacteria per pearl, laboratory assays show that these pearls actually contain 2.4 billion bacteria.

Take one Pearls Elite from Enzymatic Therapy daily for five months, after which time you may choose to continue taking one every other day for prevention. If you are on antibiotics, take acidophilus at least three to six hours before or after the antibiotic dose. Check off treatment #7 in appendix A.

You'd have to eat three gallons of yogurt to get as many healthy bacteria to the colon as one of the acidophilus or probiotic pearls contains, but yogurt can be a good adjunct remedy to help heal your gut. Choose a yogurt that is sugar-free and has live bacterial cultures (read the ingredients on the label).

Lauricidin (Monolaurin)

Monolaurin has been shown to be active against a number of viruses and bacteria, along with antifungal activity, making it an excellent way to get rid of yeast and help maintain health and improve immune function. It's produced by extracting lauric acid from coconut oil and binding it to a glycerin using a molecular distillation process. Check off treatment #7a in appendix A. You'll also find instructions for use.

PRESCRIPTION MEDICATIONS FOR YEAST OVERGROWTH

In some cases, if you still have symptoms of yeast overgrowth, such as fatigue, sinusitis, or spastic colon, you may need to take your treatment a step further. Your Holistic practitioner (information about how to find one is below) can prescribe a prescription medication such as Diflucan to more aggressively treat your yeast overgrowth. Check with your Holistic doctor about what may work best for you.

Diflucan

Diflucan (fluconazole) is a very effective prescription treatment for yeast/candida, especially if you have chronic sinusitis and/or spastic colon. After one month on the natural treatments above, add the medication Diflucan. Take 200 mg a day for six to twelve weeks. Get the generic form, fluconazole. If you have preexisting active liver disease, you should be cautious about using Diflucan or don't take it at all.

Diflucan is often also used (in a one- to three-day course) for vaginal yeast infections, which represent a small part of the overall yeast issue. A single tablet may eradicate the yeast in the vagina (and often just for a short while), but is simply not enough to eliminate the larger yeast infections in the colon, sinuses, and prostate gland.

If symptoms flare up when you take the Diflucan, stop until the symptom flare settles down. Then restart the Diflucan at just 25 to 100 mg each morning for the first three to fourteen days. If yeast symptoms (i.e., sugar craving, fatigue, sinusitis, or spastic colon) recur after you stop the Diflucan, or you feel like you are better but still have a way to go in your improvement, your holistic doctor will likely recommend that you continue taking the medication for an additional six weeks at 200 mg a day. If you experience no improvement in these symptoms, your physician may suggest another medication. If you cannot get Diflucan from your physician (Diflucan is considered a holistic treatment, so don't be surprised if your doctor is unfamiliar with using it), the rest of the program will still help, but it will not kill off the yeast in your sinuses, as the Diflucan will. Another good reason to find a holistic physician. See below.

Diflucan can be expensive, about $600 for six weeks, if you use the brand name. However, the generic form fluconazole is available. Ask your healthcare practitioner if that is suitable for you.

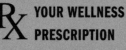
Nystatin

Nystatin, another antifungal medication, used to be effective, but more and more fungi seem to be developing resistance to it. Additionally, Nystatin is not absorbed well, which means it will not eliminate yeast outside the bowel. Because of this, I sometimes add the antifungal herbs listed previously to the Diflucan instead of Nystatin.

The antifungal medication Lamisil (used for toenail infections) is simply *not* effective for candida.

Keeping Yeast in Check

Once your symptoms of yeast overgrowth are gone, you'll feel much better. However, symptoms sometimes recur. Signs of recurrent yeast overgrowth include a return of bowel symptoms (gas, bloating, and/or diarrhea or constipation), vaginal yeast, mouth sores, and/or recurring nasal congestion or sinusitis. This may happen soon after you stop taking Diflucan, but it is more likely to occur months or even years later. It often happens after you eat too much sugar (for instance, bingeing on sugary foods during the holiday season) or after taking antibiotics.

Finding a Doctor Who Can Help Treat Candida

Unfortunately, there is no test that distinguishes normal yeast growth from overgrowth. Therefore, many conventional doctors still do not address this issue. Because of this, you may need to find a holistic physician to get the treatment you need. (See www.holisticboard.org for a list of more than two thousand board-certified holistic physicians in the United States.)

If these symptoms persist (during a recurrence) for more than two weeks, I may repeat the probiotics and antifungal herbs for one to three months. If the symptoms are severe or persistent, I may also repeat the Diflucan for six-week courses as needed. If a second round of treatment resolves the symptoms, your doctor may opt to repeat this regimen as often as needed, usually every six to twenty-four months. By using antifungal herbs and probiotic pearls, however, you may be able to avoid the need for repeated use of antifungals and the possible risk of becoming resistant to them.

Some people with very severe Candida overgrowth find that they need to stay on the antifungals for extended periods of time, years in some cases, or their symptoms recur. As an alternative, instead of taking antifungals every day, many people find they can suppress the yeast long term by taking 200 mg of Diflucan twice a day, once a week (for example, each Sunday).

IMMUNE SUPPORT FOR TYPE 3 SUGAR ADDICTS

Maintaining a healthy immune system is critical to getting rid of yeast. A strong immune system can prevent infections that might lead to excess antibiotic use, which fuels yeast overgrowth. The following nutrients are essential for keeping your body's defenses working properly:

Zinc may well be the single most important nutrient for maintaining optimal immune function. This mineral is in every cell; an antioxidant, it protects cells in the body from free radical damage, which can cause aging and may be a factor in health problems like heart disease and cancer. Chronic infections can cause large losses of zinc from the body, resulting in nutritional deficiencies. Zinc deficiency will cause marked immune suppression. Recommended daily dose: 15 to 25 mg.

Vitamin A is critical for mucosal immunity, which can help prevent respiratory and bowel infections that often accompany yeast overgrowth. Recommended daily dose: 2,000 to 3,500 IU.

Vitamin C actually does make you less likely to catch a cold. A review of the medical literature published in the *Journal of Military Medicine* in 2004 showed that in five studies participants who took vitamin C experienced a 45 to 91 percent reduction in common cold incidence. Three other trials found a marked reduction in the incidence of pneumonia in

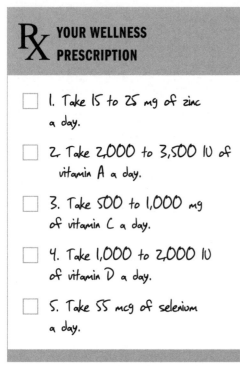

RX YOUR WELLNESS PRESCRIPTION

- [ ] 1. Take 15 to 25 mg of zinc a day.

- [ ] 2. Take 2,000 to 3,500 IU of vitamin A a day.

- [ ] 3. Take 500 to 1,000 mg of vitamin C a day.

- [ ] 4. Take 1,000 to 2,000 IU of vitamin D a day.

- [ ] 5. Take 55 mcg of selenium a day.

the vitamin C group. Recommended daily dose: 500 to 1,000 mg.

Vitamin D helps the body absorb calcium and phosphorus needed for healthy bones, but it is also especially important in regulating and supporting immune function. New research published in the *Journal of Clinical Endocrinology & Metabolism (JCEM)* in February 2014 confirmed that older people who don't get enough Vitamin D have compromised immune function, which can make them more prone to illness. Another study published in the *JCEM* in April 2014 revealed that cancer patients who have higher levels of vitamin D when they were diagnosed tended to have better survival rates and remain in remission longer than patients who were vitamin D-deficient. Vitamin D deficiency increases the risk of infections and can also increase the risk of diabetes.

Most of our vitamin D comes from sunshine, but it's estimated that more than 1 billion people worldwide just don't get enough exposure. Sunshine in moderation is fine. Just remember: Avoid sunburn, not sunshine! Supplementation can also help bridge the gap. Recommended daily dose: 1,000 to 2,000 IU.

Selenium is critical for optimal immune function. This antioxidant can help eliminate the sinusitis and bowel infections commonly seen in type 3 sugar addicts. Recommended daily dose: 55 mcg.

All of the above can be found in a good vitamin powder. (Check off treatment #1 in appendix A.)

ARE FOOD ALLERGIES AGGRAVATING YOUR SUGAR CRAVINGS?

Eliminating yeast will get rid of most food sensitivities and sugar cravings, especially if you also treat for adrenal fatigue. (See chapter 7.) For some people, though, food allergies may persist, causing fatigue, bloating after eating, runny nose, and even an increase in pulse rate after eating. Most blood tests for food allergies tend to be unreliable and can make you neurotic about what you eat. The Multiple Food Elimination Diet, which screens for food allergies, can be helpful for determining which foods you are allergic to. Avoiding these foods—or better yet, eliminating the allergies using an acupressure technique called NAET (see www.NAET.com)—can result in increased energy, decreased sugar cravings, and the elimination of digestive and many other problems.

Some yeast experts recommend avoiding all yeast-containing foods. This advice is based on the theory that an allergic reaction to yeast is the cause of the problem. However, the yeast found in most foods (except beer and cheese) is not closely related to candida, the predominant yeast that seems to be involved in overgrowth. Although a few individuals do appear to have true allergies to the yeast in their food, they account for fewer than 10 percent of people with suspected yeast overgrowth.

If you do have a yeast allergy, or especially severe candida problems, you may benefit from the more strict diet recommended in the late Dr. William Crook's book *The Yeast Connection Handbook*. Dr. Crook spent a lifetime teaching doctors about candida, and he was a giant in his field. His book, and the website www.yeastconnection.com, are excellent sources for more information.

The Multiple Food Elimination Diet for Food Allergies

Using the Multiple Food Elimination Diet created by Doris Rapp, MD, board-certified in pediatrics, allergy, and environmental medicine, clinical assistant professor of pediatrics at SUNYAB (Emeritus), and author of the *New York Times* bestseller *Is This Your Child?*, will help you discover which foods may be triggering your food allergies. If you have food allergies, you are most likely allergic to the foods you crave and eat the most. The Multiple Food Elimination Diet, however, will let you clearly identify these foods. This fast, inexpensive method of food allergy detection can sometimes provide rapid, safe relief from many chronic medical and behavioral complaints.

R℞ YOUR WELLNESS PRESCRIPTION

☐ 1. Treating candida and adrenal problems often eliminates many food allergies.

☐ 2. If problems persist, use the Multiple Food Elimination Diet for seven to ten days to see if you feel better on the diet.

☐ 3. Add a food group back to your diet every one to three days to determine which foods are causing allergic or sensitivity reactions.

☐ 4. Use NAET (muscle testing and acupressure) to test for and eliminate food sensitivities.

If you want to help your entire family, urge everyone to try the diet at the same time. Typically, several family members will note improvement in how they feel or act when this is done. But it's common to experience moderate withdrawal and worsening of symptoms and cravings when the offending foods are first eliminated. This happens because you are undergoing the withdrawal symptoms caused by *not* eating a food to which you are "addicted." Sugar could be one of them. Symptoms can include headaches, weakness, irritability, and nausea. The good news is these withdrawal symptoms usually pass after you've been on the elimination diet for seven or eight days.

The Multiple Food Elimination Allergy Diet, Part 1

Part I of this diet requires seven days of abstinence from the "forbidden" foods listed below. You may not eat these foods in any form. During this first week you'll only eat the "allowed" foods. If you feel significantly better, it suggests a problematic food was avoided during this week. Keep a food diary of exactly what you eat.

Allowed Foods

- most fruits

- most vegetables

- most meats

- oats and rice

Forbidden Foods

- milk and dairy products

- wheat products, crackers, and baked goods

- eggs

- chocolate

- peas

- peanut butter

- citrus (orange, lemon, lime, and grapefruit)

- food dyes

- additives and preservatives

- bacon and smoked meats

- most canned or prepackaged soups

If you have some question about a specific food, or if it is one of your favorites but it's not listed above, do not eat it. You'll also need to delete coffee, tea, any other highly craved foods (e.g., cinnamon or mushrooms), alcohol in any form, and tobacco because any of these can be the cause of chronic illness.

It's very likely that you will notice a big difference in how you feel by the fifth to seventh day on this diet. Although rare, some people experience improvement before the fourth day. The object is to see the maximum amount of improvement that can be noted during the first seven days. If you are feeling better within a week's time, begin Part 2 of the diet on the eighth day—or sooner if there is tremendous improvement in less than one week.

Here is a more specific list of food do's and don'ts:

ALLOWED FOODS	FORBIDDEN FOODS
Cereals—Rice (rice puffs only) and oats (oatmeal made with honey barley)	Cereals—Foods containing wheat flour (most cookies, cakes, bread, and baked goods), corn, popcorn, and cereal mixtures (e.g., granola)
Fruits—Any fresh fruit except citrus, and canned fruit if in their own juice and without artificial color, sugar, or preservatives	Fruits—Citrus (orange, lemon, lime, and grapefruit)
Vegetables—Any fresh vegetables except corn and peas; potatoes and homemade french fries	Vegetables—Any frozen or canned vegetables, corn, peas, or mixed vegetables
Meats—Chicken and turkey (non-basted), Louis Rich ground turkey, beef, pork, lamb, fish, and tuna	Meats—Luncheon meats, wieners, bacon, artificially dyed hamburger/meat, ham, dyed salmon, lobster, breaded meats, and meats with stuffing
Beverages—Water and single herb or plain tea with stevia	Beverages—Milk or dairy drinks with casein or whey, fruit beverages except those so specified, Kool-Aid, Coffee Rich (yellow dye), and all sodas and sugar-containing juice
Snacks—Potato chips (no additives), RyKrisp crackers and pure honey, and raisins (unsulfured)	Snacks—Corn chips, chocolate/cocoa, hard candy, and ice cream or sherbet
Miscellaneous—Homemade vinegar/oil dressing, sea salt, pepper, and homemade soup	Miscellaneous—Sugar, bread, cake, cookies, eggs, dyed (colored) vitamins, pills, mouthwash, toothpaste, medicines (such as cough syrups, etc.), jelly or jam, gelatin, margarine/diet spreads (with dyes and corn), peanut butter/ peanuts, Sorbitol (corn), cheese, and soy

When to Stop the Diet

Occasionally, you may feel much worse during Part 1 of the diet. If this happens, immediately stop the diet. You may have begun to ingest an excessive amount of an unsuspected offending food or beverage. A child who substitutes apple or grape juice for milk, for example, may act or behave much worse if apple or grape juice is actually the cause of this child's symptoms.

If you get an infection of some kind while you're on the diet, stop the diet until you are well. It is too difficult to interpret the results under these conditions.

Recheck Your Diet Diary and Start Again

Recheck your diet diary for the initial week of the diet. Try Part 1 of the diet again, leaving out any food or beverage that you suspect may have made you worse. Ask yourself this question: Did you eat only the allowed foods?

If you repeatedly forgot and ate the wrong foods or drank the wrong beverages, the item that was not omitted from the diet may be the culprit. Begin Part 1 of the diet again, but this time try much harder to adhere strictly to the "allowed" foods. It's best to do the diet only one time, but do it right.

When the Elimination Diet Is Not the Answer

If Part 1 of the diet has not helped you by the fourteenth day, this particular diet is probably not the answer for you. Either your medical problems are not related to food allergies or they're due to other frequently eaten or craved items that were not removed from the diet.

You may want to try NAET (Nambudripad's Allergy Elimination Techniques), an acupressure technique that lets you successfully test for food allergies and sensitivities. One twenty-minute treatment can help you eliminate one allergy. Research we've done even shows that autistic children can find relief with NAET. There are more than 12,000 practitioners worldwide (see www.NAET.com for one near you).

The Multiple Food Elimination Allergy Diet, Part 2

Once you've successfully completed the Multiple Elimination Diet for one week, it's time to go to the next step. During the next ten days of the diet, you'll be adding back previously omitted foods into your diet, one at a time. If you have an adverse reaction, such as a headache, wait until it goes away to try another eliminated food. It's best if the foods are added back into your diet in the following sequence:

- On Day 8, add milk

- On Day 9, add wheat

- On Day 10, add sugar

- On Day 11, add eggs

- On Day 12, add cocoa

- On Day 13, add food coloring

- On Day 14, add corn

- On Day 15, add preservatives

- On Day 16, add citrus

- On Day 17, add peanut butter

Eat the test food repeatedly during the day, preferably by itself. Unless the food you're testing is normally eaten in meal-size portions, it is best to start with 1 teaspoon (5 ml) or 1/2 cup (235 ml) of the item. Then double the amount you eat every few hours, so that by the end of the day you've ingested at least a normal amount. You can eat "allowed foods" as often as you'd like during the first week of Part 2 of the diet.

Adding Foods to Your Diet Day by Day

Day 8: The day you add milk, drink lots of milk and eat cottage cheese and whipped cream sweetened with honey. Avoid butter, margarine, or yellow cheese unless you are very certain they contain no yellow dyes.

Day 9: The day you add wheat, eat plain wheat cereal. If eating milk caused problems, be sure not to ingest milk products. Even crackers can contain milk. Italian bread or kosher bread usually does not contain milk (casein or whey), but always read the labels to make sure. You can bake if you like, but you must not use eggs or sugar. If milk caused no problem, milk products may be eaten on Day 9.

Day 10: The day you add sugar, eat sugar cubes. If milk or wheat caused trouble, avoid them or you won't be able to tell whether you can tolerate sugar. You will probably start to feel or act differently within one hour after consuming four to eight large sugar cubes. (Eat this higher amount of sugar just for one day as a test.)

Day 11: The day you add egg, eat eggs in the usual cooked forms. Remember, no wheat, milk, or sugar can be consumed if any of these substances caused problems. If you experienced no problems, you can eat eggs in the form of custard or an egg-white topping.

Day 12: The day you add cocoa, eat dark chocolate and cocoa. If you had no trouble with sugar and milk, you can eat milk chocolate. It's best to make hot chocolate with water, cocoa powder, and honey. No candy bars are allowed because most contain corn, plus many other ingredients. Remember, absolutely no milk, wheat, sugar, or eggs are allowed if these caused adverse reactions.

Day 13: The day you add food coloring, eat colored gelatin, jelly, or artificially colored fruit beverages (such as soda or Kool-Aid), Popsicles, or cereal. Try a variety of yellow, green, purple, and red items because you may react to only one of these food dyes. Remember to avoid milk, wheat, sugar, eggs, or cocoa if they created a problem for you. If sugar caused symptoms, use honey. If you were able to tolerate milk, wheat, sugar, eggs, and cocoa, you can continue to eat them.

Day 14: The day you add corn, eat a variety of corn products, such as whole kernel corn, cornmeal, cornflakes, corn syrup, and popcorn. Try several forms of corn because sometimes only one will cause illness. Popcorn can be air popped and eaten plain without salt, oil, or butter. If milk, wheat, sugar, eggs, dyes, or cocoa caused symptoms, you can't eat them on the same day that you introduce corn back into your diet. If you do, you won't be able to tell which food is at fault. Use butter on the popcorn only if you had no milk sensitivity.

Day 15: The day you add preservatives, eat foods that contain preservatives or food additives. Read the labels and look for foods that include the longest list of additives. In particular, eat luncheon meat, bologna, hot dogs, breads, pastries, or soups that contain numerous preservatives and additives.

Day 16: The day you add citrus, eat a large amount of lemon, lime, grapefruit, or orange as fresh fruit and/or as a juice. Avoid artificial dyes if food colorings were a problem or citrus drinks because they usually contain other ingredients. Avoid regular gelatin or gelatin-like preparations if sugar or dyes were a problem for you. Instead, buy plain gelatin and make your own with pure fruit juice and honey. Use carbonated water in pure juice to create homemade "soda." Do not consume beverages with aspartame, saccharin, sucralose, or Sucaryl because they can also cause symptoms in some individuals.

Day 17: The day you add peanut butter, eat lots of pure peanut butter without additives or plain peanuts. Test for this only if it's a favorite food. Eat the peanut butter from the spoon or put it on RyKrisp crackers or rice cakes if you experienced problems with wheat.

Pinpointing Offending Foods

Keep detailed records of how you feel, before and after the test food is eaten. If symptoms occur within an hour (or that same day, or by the next morning), it could indicate that the test food is causing the problem.

- Do any symptoms suddenly reappear within an hour after eating the test food for that day?

- Do any symptoms gradually reappear as the day progresses, after you've eaten more and more of the test food for that day?

If you experience no undesirable symptoms during that day, during that night, and the next morning before breakfast, the food tested the day before is probably all right and you may eat it whenever you desire.

If you react to any food, ingesting the following can help, usually in twenty minutes or less:

- Tri-Salts (available at health food stores), 1 to 2 teaspoons in 1/2 to 1 cup (235 ml) of water

- Sodium bicarbonate (baking soda), 1 to 2 teaspoons in 1/2 to 1 cup (235 ml) of water

- Alka-Aid (available at health food stores), 1/2 to 2 tablets

- Also use an antihistamine or asthma medicine if needed. If a reaction is severe, go to the nearest doctor or emergency room.

If a test food reaction is not mitigated by the above or lasts for more than twenty-four hours, do not try to check the response to another possible problem food until the previous food reaction has entirely subsided.

Watch closely to see what happens each day because each food might cause a different response. For instance, one food might cause abdominal pain, another might cause stuffiness in your head or sinuses, and another might produce no reaction at all. Most reactions occur within fifteen to sixty minutes; others, within several hours.

If you are uncertain whether a food truly caused symptoms or not, discontinue that food until the other foods have been checked. Then, ingest that particular suspect food again at a four-day interval, for example, on Tuesday and Saturday, to see whether the same symptoms recur.

Never test any food without your doctor's advice if it caused serious medical problems for you in the past. For example, if eating egg, corn, or peanut caused immediate throat swelling, it is unsafe to try even a speck of these foods. The purpose of the diet is to find out what you don't know or to confirm questions about suspicious foods, not to make yourself ill or to cause a life-threatening allergic reaction. Additional details are available in Doris Rapp's book, *Allergies and Your Family.*

Using NAET to Eliminate Food and Sugar Sensitivities

NAET, developed by Devi S. Nambudripad, MD, PhD, DC, LAc, RN, is a powerful yet gentle cutting-edge technique that lets you successfully test for food allergies and sensitivities. It uses muscle testing to determine what you are sensitive to, then employs acupressure to quickly eliminate one sensitivity or allergy with each twenty-minute treatment. There are more than 12,000 practitioners worldwide (see www.NAET.com for one near you).

Most sugar addicts also have sensitivities to other foods and substances. NAET desensitizes your addictions to sugar and carbohydrates, enabling you to stop craving sugar by teaching your body to digest, absorb, and assimilate sugar from your food intake. Once this has been accomplished, food allergies and sensitivities can be tested for and eliminated. After seven to ten treatment sessions of about twenty minutes each, a patient usually begins seeing benefits. Eliminating most food allergies in most sugar addicts takes between fifteen and thirty sessions.

I was a very skeptical physician when I first heard about the technique. Basically, I thought it was silly—until a single twenty-minute treatment immediately eliminated my lifelong and severe ragweed pollen allergy (hay fever). It was like someone turned off a faucet in my nose. Medically, this was not supposed to happen, but it did. My mind finally opened, and I flew to California to meet Dr. Nambudripad. She is an amazing woman with many degrees, a great heart, and no ego. I then married the wonderful woman back home who had treated me. (I guess I must have been very impressed!)

Summary: An Action Plan for Type 3 Sugar Addicts

1. Treat yeast overgrowth by changing your diet: eliminating processed sugar and white flour. (Dark chocolate is the one exception.)

2. Use the sugar substitutes stevia, PureVia, or Truvia.

3. Treat your yeast overgrowth with probiotics and anti-yeast herbs.

4. If you have a severe yeast overgrowth, ask your holistic doctor to prescribe the prescription medicine Diflucan.

5. Use a vitamin powder to provide optimal nutritional support.

6. Boost immunity with key vitamins and minerals, including zinc and vitamin C.

7. If you have chronic sinusitis or spastic colon, see part III.

8. If you have food allergies, try the Multiple Food Elimination Diet by Dr. Doris Rapp. You may also find NAET to be especially helpful.

9. Check off treatments #1, #6, and #7 in appendix A.

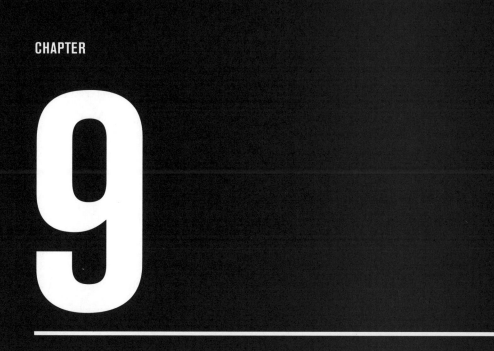

CHAPTER

9

TREATMENT FOR TYPE 4 SUGAR ADDICTS: REBALANCE HORMONAL FLUCTUATIONS

When hormones go wacky during PMS, perimenopause, menopause, or andropause (male menopause), they can cause sugar cravings to soar. These conditions can lead to insulin resistance, which makes it difficult for your body to control blood sugar levels and make you feel tired, irritable, and miserable when you eat sweets. In order to stop type 4 sugar addiction, you'll need to take a whole body approach to treating hormonal imbalances. By combining a healthy diet, bio-identical hormones, and/or natural remedies, you can heal your body and feel better than ever before.

Your treatment program includes the following steps:

1. Make simple dietary changes to stop sugar addiction.

2. Use natural remedies to heal your body, ease symptoms, and treat sugar addiction.

3. Use bio-identical hormones if needed to treat hormonal deficiencies and curb sugar cravings.

YOUR WELLNESS PRESCRIPTION

- [ ] 1. Avoid foods high in sugar.

- [ ] 2. Avoid white flour.

- [ ] 3. Eat foods that score low on the glycemic index.

- [ ] 4. Eat high-protein foods.

- [ ] 5. Choose organic foods whenever possible.

- [ ] 6. Stay hydrated.

- [ ] 7. For women in menopause, eat a handful of soybean pods (edamame) each day.

- [ ] 8. Supplement with key nutrients.

- [ ] 9. Exercise for thirty to sixty minutes a day, outside if possible.

A DIET PLAN FOR TYPE 4 SUGAR ADDICTS

Simple dietary changes can make a big difference in the way you feel, whether you have PMS or are in perimenopause, menopause, or andropause. Adjusting your diet using the wellness prescription here will help decrease insulin resistance as well as reduce your risk of diabetes, high cholesterol, and heart disease and leave you feeling much better. Eating a balanced diet and listening to your body will ensure optimal health and help you kick your sugar addiction.

Curb That Sweet Tooth

Start by getting rid of high-sugar foods in your diet, especially fast food, processed food, sodas, and fruit drinks. Make it a habit to read labels. As a rule of thumb, if sugar in any form (sugar, sucrose, glucose, fructose, or corn syrup) is one of the top three ingredients listed, don't eat that food. The one exception to the no sugar rule is dark chocolate (more about this in the sidebar). You'll also want to avoid (though not strictly) the white flour found in bread, pasta, and pizza because this is rapidly turned into sugar in your body, giving you a sugar high followed by a big low.

Eat protein, veggies, and fruit for breakfast and eat more complex carbohydrates (such as whole wheat) as the day goes on. This will help you manage sugar swings and stabilize your blood sugar. The diet for type 4 sugar addicts does not have to be as strict as with other types. Although these guidelines can help, it's important to learn to eat what leaves you feeling the best overall.

Choose Foods That Score Low on the Glycemic Index

Instead of choosing high-sugar foods or those that contain white flour, get in the habit of eating foods with low glycemic index (GI) scores, including whole grains, fruits, and vegetables. When you eat low GI foods that are digested slowly, your blood sugar will rise gradually, preventing that sugar roller coaster ride. Another way to keep your blood sugar stable and stem sugar addiction is to eat high-protein foods—think fish, chicken, turkey, cheese, and eggs.

Women in menopause who have low estrogen can benefit from eating a handful of soybean pods (edamame) daily; perimenopausal women may find eating edamame helpful around your periods. Traditionally, menopausal Japanese women have eaten a handful of edamame each day to prevent symptoms. It's a good source of natural estrogen. You'll also get a host of vitamins, minerals, and fiber from them, too. And they taste good.

Satisfy Your Sweet Tooth with Dark Chocolate

Chocolate in moderation—especially dark chocolate—offers many benefits. Chocolate contains PEA (phenylethylamine), a potent mood elevator and antidepressant. For some people, chocolate can be as effective as Prozac but without the side effects. Chocolate also contains a mild stimulant called theobromine—it gives you an energy boost, but not enough to get you on the sugar roller coaster the way caffeine does. Women intuitively crave chocolate because they know it is good for them and improves their moods. It's okay to eat up to a few ounces (85 to 115 g) a day, especially if you're feeling down or depressed.

They can be found in the frozen vegetable section in most supermarkets, or ask at your health food store. Eating large amounts of other soy products, such as soymilk and soy cheese, is not a good alternative because these tend to block thyroid hormone function.

Drink Water to Support Hormonal Function

As with other sugar addiction types, it's very important for people in perimenopause, menopause, or andropause to drink enough water. Water helps the machinery of the body function and lets the body rid itself of toxins. How much water should you drink a day? Check your mouth and lips every so often. If they are dry, you are thirsty and need to drink more water. It's that simple.

But drinking tap water isn't the way to go. Tap water's great for cleaning dishes and clothes, but not so good for routine human consumption. Tap water just isn't as pure as it should be and can be full of chemicals that can interfere with estrogen, progesterone, and testosterone function. Bottled water has problems, too. Many brands of bottled water are simply tap water, and cost has little to do with quality. But we need to have easy access to healthy water. So how can you tell what is best?

When drinking bottled water, use water that is purified by reverse osmosis and carbon block filtration. For home use, a good-quality water filter is best (see "Water Filters" in appendix D for more information). When you're on the go, carry filtered water in glass or stainless steel bottles—the hormone-blocking chemicals in plastic bottles can leach into the water.

Why Choose Organic Foods?

Organic fruits and vegetables are grown without toxic insecticides and pesticides that can interfere with the normal function of hormones in your body. Organic meat (ideally humanely raised too) comes from animals that aren't fed artificial hormones or diets that contain synthetic additives. Organic food is grown in rich soil, full of nutrients, as opposed to the depleted soils caused by traditional farming methods. If you can't afford to buy all organic products, at least choose organic varieties of the foods you eat most often.

Nutritional Supplements for Type 4 Sugar Addicts

Optimizing nutritional support with specific vitamins helps you kick type 4 sugar addiction in many ways. First, you'll find the additional nutrients decrease the anxiety and depression you may have that can drive sugar addiction. Certain supplements can also help decrease the risk of osteoporosis, which increases with estrogen deficiency and antidepressant use. In fact, nutritional support is far more effective than medications for treating both depression and osteoporosis. In part III, we'll discuss treatment for both of these conditions, which are common in type 4 sugar addicts.

Begin with a foundation of a good vitamin and mineral powder. (Check off treatment #1 in appendix A.) Taking a vitamin powder is an easy and effective way to get the many nutrients you need to address deficiencies you may have as a type 4 sugar addict and to support overall good health. In addition, it's especially important to supplement with vitamin B_1, vitamin B_{12}, and iodine (present in the powder).

Vitamin B_1 decreases both anxiety and depression, and it is critical for proper brain functioning. Research published in the medical journal *Psychopharmacology* in 1997 showed that supplementation with vitamin B_1 improves mood, possibly by increasing the synthesis of acetylcholine. This neurotransmitter is associated with memory and also makes you more clearheaded, composed, and energetic. Recommended daily dose: 75 mg.

Vitamin B_{12} helps not only depression but also mood in general. Research published in the *International Journal of Neuropsychopharmacology* in 2005 showed that when people are treated for depression, those with higher levels of vitamin B_{12} tend to get a greater benefit from antidepressants. This may be due to the fact that a deficiency in vitamin B_{12} can result in high homocysteine levels, which may enhance depression. Recommended daily dose: 500 mcg.

Iodine deficiency contributes not only to fatigue but also to breast cysts and the breast tenderness that often accompanies PMS. Research on breast cancer rates in Japanese women found them to be two-thirds lower than in American women. It is suspected that this may be due to the high Japanese intake of seaweed, which is rich in iodine. Recommended daily dose: 150+ mcg.

How Can Vitamin D and Exercise Help Type 4 Sugar Addicts?

Not getting enough vitamin D can increase the risk of depression, which can exacerbate sugar cravings. More than 90 percent of our vitamin D comes from sunshine. So avoid sunburn, but not sunshine.

Exercise is also important for type 4 sugar addicts. By raising the happiness molecule serotonin and the "runner's high" brain chemical endorphin, exercise helps alleviate depression and mood shifts. Taking a daily walk or enjoying another form of exercise outdoors in the sunshine provides the added benefits of vitamin D. The combination eases the anxiety and depression caused by reproductive hormone deficiencies--and the sugar cravings that go along with them.

NATURAL REMEDIES FOR TREATING PMS

As you learned in chapter 4, PMS is associated with increased anxiety, moodiness, bloating, and depression around your menstrual period. This triggers sugar cravings as your body tries to use sugar to raise the "happiness molecule" serotonin and help you feel better. In time, though, eating sugar becomes counterproductive and just makes your symptoms worse.

Although there is significant controversy about the cause of PMS, it appears to be associated with low levels of the hormones progesterone and prostaglandin E1 and E3. These hormone deficiencies have been linked with anxiety, moodiness, and generally feeling less than your best. The wellness prescription below will cut your sugar cravings and help you feel better in general.

Note: It takes three months to get the full benefit of these remedies for PMS, though you may start to see results more quickly. If you are on birth control pills and your symptoms hit when you stop the pill for a week each month, ask your doctor if you can take the pill every day without stopping it. Let your doctor know you have PMS so s/he can adjust the brand of pill if necessary. The FDA has approved birth control pills (e.g., Seasonale) that can be stopped only one week every three months, instead of one week each month.

℞ YOUR WELLNESS PRESCRIPTION

☐ 1. Take 50 mg of vitamin B₆ a day.

☐ 2. Take 3,000 mg of evening primrose oil or borage oil a day for three months, then just during the week before your period.

☐ 3. Eat salmon or tuna three or more times a week. You can also supplement with a high quality fish oil that contains omega 3 essential fatty acids.

☐ 4. Take 200 to 400 mg of magnesium daily.

☐ 5. Take 50 to 200 mg of theanine one to three times a day as needed for anxiety or to help sleep.

☐ 6. Take one-half to one scoop of a good multivitamin powder each day, long term.

☐ 7. If PMS is still problematic after three months, add 200 mg of prescription natural progesterone at bedtime. Take two 100 mg capsules by mouth (Prometrium can be found at most pharmacies) or compounded progesterone cream 30 mg topically daily for the week before your period (30 mg applied to the skin is equal to 100 mg taken by mouth).

☐ 8. Check off treatments #1, 4, and 8 (and if symptoms persist, #10) in appendix A.

☐ 9. If anxiety and depression persist, see part III.

Take Vitamin B₆ to Reduce Irritability and Sugar Cravings

Vitamin B_6 is important if you have PMS because it eases the deficiency of the "feel good" hormone prostaglandin E1. When this hormone is low, irritability and sugar cravings can result. Take 50 mg of extra vitamin B_6 a day for three to six months—it even helps relieve fluid retention in your hands and fingers.

After taking the extra dose of vitamin B_6 for three to six months, the amount contained in the vitamin powder will usually be plenty. Cutting out sugar and increasing your overall nutritional support will allow your body to recover.

Take Evening Primrose Oil to Aid Sugar-Related Depression

Your body uses the oils found in your diet for many different purposes, the most important being to make hormones called prostaglandins. These hormones are critical for controlling inflammation and mood. Prostaglandin E1 (PGE1), made from the essential fatty acid gamma-linolenic acid (GLA), is found in certain vegetable oils. GLA is then converted into dihomo-gamma-linolenic acid (DGLA), which then is turned into prostaglandin E1. Unfortunately, excess sugar and nutritional deficiencies (especially vitamin B_6 and magnesium) block your ability to turn the GLA in vegetable oils into DGLA, causing prostaglandin E1 deficiency, which leads to depression. Eating sugar causes a brief mood elevation, but then worsens your hormone deficiency.

Cutting out sugar allows your body to make prostaglandin more effectively. The "chemical blockade" caused by sugar excess can also be bypassed by taking DGLA directly. This oil is found in high amounts in evening primrose oil (expensive) or borage oil (cheaper). Take 3,000 mg a day of evening primrose oil for three months, after which time you can take the oil just during the week before your period. (Efamol is a good brand.) Once you are feeling better, you can switch to less expensive borage oil and see whether it works as well for you. Most people find that the borage oil works fine; if cost is a factor, it's okay to simply start with borage oil.

Take Fish Oil to Elevate Your Mood

Fish oil improves your mood in general and depression specifically. The essential fatty acids in fish oil help make mood-elevating prostaglandin PGE3. Fish oil has been shown in numerous studies to aid depression as well as many other psychological problems. In the May 1999 *Archives of General Psychiatry*, Andrew Stoll, MD, and colleagues reported a study in which 10 grams of fish oil a day markedly improved symptoms in 64 percent of manic-depressive patients after four months (versus only 19 percent of those receiving the placebo). Joseph Hibbeln, MD, a psychiatrist at the National Institutes of Health, thinks fish oil deficiency might explain why the rate of depression is rising in the United States.

In addition, taking fish oil during pregnancy markedly decreases the risk of postpartum depression. Postpartum depression is very similar to the symptoms of PMS because both conditions are related to progesterone deficiencies. A deficiency of the hormone progesterone causes sugar cravings. Eating coldwater fish, such as salmon and mackerel, which are rich in omega-3 essential fatty acids, can decrease postpartum depression by half. You can also take a tablespoon (15 ml) of a mercury-free fish oil a day to ease symptoms.

If you are depressed, try eating three or more servings of salmon, tuna, or herring each week and/or supplement with fish oil, Omega 3. (Check off treatment #8 in appendix A for Evening Primrose oil and fish oil.) The best way to do this is to take one or two Vectomega tablets (EuroPharma) a day. This replaces 8–16 fish oil capsules. Another benefit? Fish oil decreases arthritis and heart disease risk.

Most of your brain is actually made of DHA (docosahexaenoic acid), one of the two key components of fish oil. Fish is called "brain food" for a good reason. You'll learn more about treating depression in part III.

Take Magnesium to Relieve Stress and Sugar Cravings

Magnesium has been called the "anti-stress mineral." Magnesium relaxes muscles, improves sleep, and relieves tension. Like vitamin B_6, magnesium increases the production of PGE1, so it eases the deficiency of prostaglandin E1 that causes irritability and drives sugar cravings. Magnesium also helps make the three key "happiness" neurotransmitters that your body needs: serotonin, dopamine, and norepinephrine.

Take Theanine to Reduce Anxiety

If you experience anxiety related to PMS, theanine—which comes from green tea—can help. Theanine stimulates your body's production of "natural Valium," called gamma-aminobutyric acid (GABA), without addiction or side effects. It will keep you calm and alert during the day, while helping you sleep at night. Theanine also naturally stimulates the release of the "happiness molecules" serotonin and dopamine. In addition, theanine increases alpha brain wave activity, creating a state of deep relaxation and mental alertness similar to what is achieved through meditation. Check off treatment #10 for anxiety in appendix A.

Prescription Help for PMS

If PMS symptoms are still problematic after three months, ask your physician to prescribe natural progesterone (Prometrium). Take one to two 100 mg capsules by mouth or use 30 mg of compounded progesterone cream topically daily for the week before your period. It is okay to begin it as soon as PMS symptoms seem to begin.

Prometrium can be found in most standard pharmacies, and it is usually covered by prescription insurance. It is natural and bio-identical. We advise against using the synthetic progesterone called Provera, which many studies suggest is horribly toxic.

TREATING PROBLEMS DUE TO PERIMENOPAUSE AND MENOPAUSE

The estrogen and progesterone deficiency that happens in menopause actually begins in perimenopause, five to twelve years before your blood tests become abnormal (i.e., FSH and LH levels go very high) and your period stops. You can tell whether you are in perimenopause if symptoms such as fatigue, anxiety, sadness, depression, insomnia, and headache are worse around your period. Other symptoms include vaginal dryness and sweats/hot flashes that worsen in the week before your period.

These symptoms are often accompanied by marked sugar cravings. Proper treatment can not only curb your sugar cravings but can also leave you feeling and looking years younger than your actual age.

Rx YOUR WELLNESS PRESCRIPTION

☐ 1. For hot flashes: Take the herb Black Cohosh (Remifemin): two capsules twice a day for two months and then reduce the dose to one capsule twice a day. Check off treatment #9 in appendix A. Also eat a handful of edamame (soybean pods) each day for a natural estrogen boost.

☐ 2. For depression caused by low estrogen: Take the herbs magnolia (30 to 90 mg of the extract a day) and St. John's wort (900 mg a day) and supplement with the amino acid 5-HTP (up to 300 mg a day—less if on prescription antidepressants). Check off treatment #17 in appendix A. Eat salmon or tuna at least three or four times a week.

☐ 3. For anxiety caused by low progesterone: Take 30 to 200 mg of natural progesterone a day.

☐ 4. For sleep dysfunction: Take wild lettuce, lemon balm, hops, theanine, valerian, or passionflower. Magnesium and/or melatonin can also be helpful.

☐ 5. Use bio-identical hormones to treat estrogen and progesterone deficiencies to improve energy, libido, and overall well-being. Try bio-identical hormone cream from a compounding pharmacy (a mixture of 0.3 to 2.5 mg of Biest plus 30 to 50 mg of progesterone is a common dose). After the first month, add 1/2 to 2 mg of testosterone to the cream if testosterone levels are low or low normal.

☐ 6. If severe fatigue, insomnia, and achiness persist, see chapter 11 for Chronic Fatigue/Fibromyalgia treatments.

Natural Remedies for Menopausal Complaints

The number one herbal remedy for menopausal problems, particularly hot flashes, is black cohosh, specifically Remifemin by Enzymatic Therapy. Study after study shows that the only brand that works for menopause symptoms is Remifemin, including a placebo-controlled study published in the journal *Obstetrics and Gynecology* in 2005.

Mark Blumenthal, founder and executive director of the American Botanical Council (the most respected source for information on herbs in the United States), noted, "Remifemin is clearly the world's most clinically tested black cohosh product, with over fifteen clinical trials that demonstrate the safety and efficacy of the product." Yale University School of Medicine clinical professor Mary Jane Minkin, MD, also recommends Remifemin as a standard alternative to hormone replacement therapy (HRT). Remifemin is also safe for women with a history of breast cancer who cannot take estrogen.

Remifemin helps stabilize autonomic functions, including blood pressure, pulse, and sweating. This decreases hot flashes associated with low estrogen. Contrary to some misconceptions, black cohosh contains no estrogen.

When the autonomic function is balanced, you can get off the sugar roller coaster. As your energy increases, you'll be less likely to reach for sugar to artificially boost your energy. Take two capsules twice a day for two months and then reduce the dose to one capsule twice a day. Check off treatment #9 in appendix A.

Natural remedies can also aid sleep problems associated with menopause, so you're more energetic and feel less need for sugar. Wild lettuce, lemon balm, hops, theanine, valerian, passionflower, magnesium, and melatonin are some effective herbs and supplements. You can find the first six of these herbs in combination products. (Check off treatment #3 in appendix A.) Even the scent of a lavender sachet placed near your pillow can help you sleep better.

Soybean pods (called edamame) are a good natural estrogen source, and eating a handful a day is a tasty snack and can be very helpful. Edamame can be found in supermarkets in the frozen vegetable section. As with peas, throw away the pod and eat only the seeds on the inside.

Common causes of sweats and/or hot flashes include having low blood sugar while you're sleeping. Simply eating a high-protein snack (such a few slices of turkey) just before bedtime will also prevent your blood sugar from dropping while you sleep and may alleviate the problem.

Inhalation of acid reflux (especially at night while sleeping) can also cause sweating. Autonomic dysfunction as well as poor digestion can trigger reflux. To remedy this problem, take Pepcid or Tagamet at bedtime for a few nights. If the sweats markedly decrease, they are being caused by acid reflux. You'll learn more about how to treat indigestion in part III.

The onset of an underactive thyroid is common around menopause and often causes symptoms blamed on low estrogen. If your symptoms include weight gain or cold intolerance (as opposed to hot flashes), you may have an underactive thyroid—which is easy to treat. (See chapter 15.)

Why Women Gain Weight During Menopause

A woman's brain uses estrogen to balance food intake with energy output—and to tell fat where to go. After menopause, this balance is disrupted and women gain weight and in the wrong places, shifting from the hips and saddlebags to the abdomen, the most dangerous place for fat, the kind that is linked to heart disease and diabetes, say researchers at the University of Cincinnati. Bio-identical hormone replacement can reduce a menopausal woman's tendency to gain weight and provide other benefits like improved energy, sleep, and perhaps anti-aging.

BIO-IDENTICAL HORMONES CAN BALANCE DEFICIENCIES AND CURB SUGAR CRAVINGS

Many people going through midlife hormonal changes—men and women alike—develop fatigue, poor libido, and/or depression. Natural hormone replacement can improve low estrogen and progesterone levels in women and low testosterone in men and help you to feel younger. Using bio-identical hormones to treat estrogen, progesterone, and testosterone deficiencies can help boost energy, libido, and overall well-being.

Using bio-identical hormones will also help curb sugar cravings. That's because reproductive hormone deficiencies are often accompanied by anxiety and depression, which trigger sugar cravings and addiction. Treating these hormone deficiencies makes it much easier to eliminate excess sweets from your diet.

As we've discussed in chapter 4, although synthetic versions of hormones used in HRT (hormone replacement therapy) have been proven to be harmful according to the recent Women's Health Initiative study, and other research (see sidebar), bio-identical hormones do not carry the same risks as the synthetics or pregnant horse urine estrogens (like Premarin). More than eighty medical studies show that HRT with bioidentical hormones are safer and far superior to Premarin and Provera with better outcomes and fewer risks and side effects. You'll find the studies on my website here: http://www.vitality101.com/health-a-z/Menopause-safety_effectiveness_bioidentical_hormones.

Synthetic Hormones and Breast Cancer

The Nurses' Health Study followed 58,000 postmenopausal women for 16 years (725,000 person-years). Researchers found that compared with women who never used hormones, use of unopposed postmenopausal estrogen from ages 50 to 60 years increased the risk of breast cancer to age 70 by 23 percent. When progestin was added to estrogen replacement, it resulted in a tripling of the risk of breast cancer to a 67 percent increase in the risk of breast cancer! Other research shows that Provera, especially, increases breast cell proliferation, which means a higher risk of breast cancer. Natural progesterone, on the other hand, has a strong anti-proliferate effect on breast tissue.

Medical studies, such as the one by Fitzpatrick and colleagues in the *Journal of Women's Health and Gender-Based Medicine* in 2000, confirm that women report increased satisfaction when they switch from MPA (synthetic progesterones like Provera) to natural progesterone, and they enjoy an improved quality of life.

When low estrogen symptoms cannot be adequately controlled with the treatments we've discussed above, it may be worth a trial of a bio-identical estrogen called Biest, which is available from compounding pharmacies. A common dose is 1.25 to 2.5 mg daily (containing 0.25 to 0.50 mg of estradiol and 1 to 2 mg of estriol). Some women do well even on very low doses of Biest, such as 0.2 mg a day. Estriol is normally present in the body and rises during pregnancy and is protective against breast cancer. Estradiol is the other major estrogen hormone and is the form found in estrogen patches.

To prevent uterine cancer, you must also take natural progesterone when taking estrogen. As an added benefit, progesterone improves sleep and decreases anxiety. Take 30 to 200 mg a day, at bedtime. Higher doses can aggravate depression, so it's important to pay attention to how you feel and adjust the dose as needed, with your doctor's help. If you are in perimenopause, after six to nine months of taking progesterone your period will sometimes stop, especially if the hormones are taken every day instead of being cycled.

TREATING PROBLEMS DUE TO LOW TESTOSTERONE IN MEN AND WOMEN

You can think of testosterone as a kind of fountain of youth hormone for both men and, to a lesser degree, women. If you don't have enough testosterone, it can lead to fatigue and low libido, and you may feel like you are just trudging through life. When you supplement safely with this hormone, it can lead to increased energy, vitality, and well-being.

Treating Hormonal Problems Due to Andropause

If you are a healthy man entering andropause and have suboptimal testosterone levels, bio-identical, natural testosterone can help keep you very young, very late into your life. Testosterone deficiency can cause many problems, including fatigue, depression, low stamina, osteoporosis, muscle wasting, diabetes, high cholesterol, weight gain, and poor libido.

Research such as a 2006 study published in the *Archives of Internal Medicine* and other studies show that optimized levels of testosterone in men are associated with the following:

- Decreased the risk of heart disease

- Improved insulin sensitivity

- Improved muscle mass

- Improved libido and sexual function

- Decreased depression

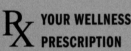

℞ YOUR WELLNESS PRESCRIPTION

☐ 1. If you are under age fifty, take 25 mg clomiphene three nights a week.

☐ 2. If you are over fifty, apply 25 to 50 mg of testosterone cream topically each day. Rub the cream into an area of thin skin on the abdomen or inner thigh.

Treating with Testosterone Is Safe

You may have heard false information about testosterone that has stopped you from adding it to your health regime. It's important to note that treatment with testosterone in men has *not* been shown to increase prostate size or the blood test marker for prostate cancer (PSA). In fact, a review of eighteen studies published in the *Journal of Urology* in 1998 showed that testosterone treatment does not increase the risk of prostate cancer. Researchers from one of the most definitive studies on testosterone published in the *Journal of the National Cancer Institute* (February 2008) stated that they found a "lack of evidence to support an androgen [testosterone]-prostate cancer hypothesis."

Testosterone used properly also does not cause heart attacks; in fact, it helps reverse heart disease when present and lowers cholesterol levels. It also improves insulin sensitivity, which means better blood sugar (glucose) control in diabetics as well as decreasing a major cause of heart disease and diabetes called «metabolic syndrome.»

Note: Don't confuse taking safe levels of bio-identical natural testosterone with the

The Wrong Ways to Boost Testosterone

Don't take testosterone pills—doing so can increase cholesterol levels. Why? Testosterone, when taken by mouth, goes to the liver first, which is where cholesterol is made. Nix injections as well because this results in very high levels of testosterone for the first few days and very low levels a week later. However, newer injections that can slowly release testosterone over several months have been developed and will offer a good option. See your holistic practitioner for more information.

high-dose, synthetic, toxic testosterone that bodybuilders sometimes use. In addition, very high doses given to men over seventy years old may unmask heart disease.

If you are under fifty, it may be best to stimulate your body's own production of testosterone using a low dose of a medication called clomiphene. A "Clomiphene Stimulation Test" will tell you whether this will work for you. Details can be found at www.vitality101.com.

If you are over fifty, use a topical testosterone cream or gel. Get Testim or Androgel from a standard pharmacy if it's covered by your prescription insurance. If not, have it made by a compounding pharmacy (50 mg testosterone plus 2.5 mg progesterone per gram of cream), which is less expensive. Always wash your hands after applying the cream. Contact with testosterone cream can cause unsafe levels in a woman's body.

Testosterone Support for Women

Although testosterone levels are normally much lower in women than in men, a deficiency can cause health problems in women as well as in men. To treat this, use a natural testosterone cream made by a compounding pharmacy. If you also need estrogen or progesterone, all three of these hormones can be combined in the same cream. Using these treatments sometimes results in more energy, thicker hair, younger-looking skin, and improved libido. Your holistic practitioner can prescribe what is right for you.

℞ YOUR WELLNESS PRESCRIPTION

☐ 1. Apply 1 to 2 mg of testosterone cream a day to your skin.

☐ 2. If needed, use a combination estrogen, progesterone, and testosterone cream.

Maintaining Proper Levels of Testosterone

You'll probably feel your best when your testosterone blood level is around the seventieth percentile of the normal range. To find out what is best for you (everyone is different), you'll need to have your testosterone levels monitored every few months. Your holistic doctor will adjust your medication accordingly.

Monitoring blood levels is especially important if you have hypothyroidism. In men, testosterone supplementation may increase levels of thyroid hormone in those taking thyroid hormone supplements, leaving you with a racing heart or anxious, hyper feelings.

Men will need a testosterone level test, complete blood count (CBC), cholesterol test, and liver enzyme test. It is important to check the free, or unbound, blood testosterone level (the active form of the hormone) in both men and women. Have your doctor adjust the testosterone level to the dose that makes you feel best within the normal range.

If you develop acne, then the dose of testosterone is too high. Testosterone can also be converted into two other hormones: estrogen and DHT (dihydrotestosterone). This can lead to bigger breasts (not a good thing if you are a man) or decreased erections (ditto!). For this reason, your doctor may also check your estrogen levels during treatment. If you have too much estrogen, you'll want to add a medication called Arimidex (0.33 mg every other day). Arimidex blocks the conversion of testosterone into estrogen. If you have problems with slow urination or a worsening of male pattern baldness associated with an increase in DHT levels, take the herb saw palmetto (160 mg twice daily) or the medication Proscar (5 mg or ½ tab) every other day along with the testosterone.

Women, if you experience acne or intense dreams or your facial hair gets darker, decrease your dose. These symptoms are usually caused by an imbalance between estrogen and testosterone. To decrease the risk of side effects, begin the estrogen four to eight weeks before starting testosterone.

Summary: An Action Plan for Type 4 Sugar Addicts

1. Avoid foods high in sugar and white flour.

2. Choose whole grains, high-protein foods, and foods that score low on the glycemic index. For PMS, add a handful of edamame a day.

3. Exercise for thirty to sixty minutes a day, outside if possible.

4. Sunshine in moderation is good for you—get thirty to sixty minutes a day.

5. Use nutritional supplements for problematic symptoms and sugar cravings related to PMS, perimenopause, menopause, or andropause.

6. Use bio-identical hormones to address hormonal deficiencies and stop sugar cravings.

7. For help with anxiety and depression, see part III.

8. Check off treatment #1 in appendix A. For PMS, check off treatments #4 and #8 (and #10 if needed for anxiety). For Menopause and Perimenopause, check off treatments #3 (as needed) and #9.

PART 3

TREATING THE SIDE EFFECTS OF SUGAR ADDICTION

In part II, you learned specific treatments for your sugar addiction type. But it's important to keep in mind that sugar addiction can be complicated. It can lead to many common and often severe problems, which must be treated if you're going to regain optimum health. Some of these problems are simply uncomfortable while others can be life threatening. These include (but aren't limited to) anxiety, chronic fatigue syndrome and fibromyalgia, depression, diabetes, heart disease, hypothyroidism, irritable bowel syndrome and spastic colon, indigestion, migraines and tension headaches, obesity, osteoporosis, and sinusitis. In part III, you'll learn about these illnesses caused by sugar addiction and how to treat them using the best natural and prescription therapies.

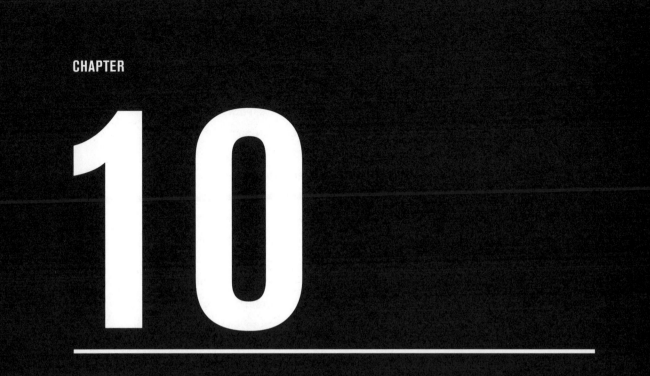

CHAPTER

10

ANXIETY

It's common for sugar addicts to suffer from anxiety. That's because sugar wreaks havoc on the central nervous system and can leave you feeling on edge. Excessive sugar intake, especially when associated with chronic stress, can also exhaust your stress-handler adrenal glands, as occurs in type 2 sugar addiction. This causes wild swings in your blood sugar levels. As levels plummet, the brain reacts by sending out a panicked adrenaline alarm, leading to severe anxiety. Over a period of years, this can become chronic.

The empty calories that sugar pumps into your diet can produce nutritional deficiencies, especially of the B vitamins and magnesium. Because B vitamins and magnesium have a relaxing effect on your system, a deficiency can intensify your response to stress and increase your anxiety.

In addition, progesterone stimulates your body's "natural Valium" (called GABA, or gamma-aminobutyric acid). Progesterone levels drop around a woman's period and decline as she begins to enter menopause. This progesterone deficiency can also trigger anxiety.

If you follow the recommendations in chapter 7 regarding treatment for type 2 sugar addiction and in chapter 9 on remedying type 4 sugar addiction, much of your anxiety will dissipate. Some of you, though, may be left with persistent anxiety because you are so accustomed to living in a heightened state of preparedness and fear. Your anxiety has become chronic. In this chapter, you'll learn about many natural treatments that can help alleviate the symptoms of anxiety.

RELIEF FROM SUGAR-RELATED ANXIETY

Anxiety can be devastating, especially when it becomes chronic and interferes with your day-to-day functioning. Unfortunately, many anxiety sufferers are simply given medications such as Valium and antidepressants to reduce their symptoms. In some cases, these medications are ineffective and can have lots of unpleasant side effects, in addition to being addictive. Furthermore, they don't resolve the problem; they just mask it.

A better way is to use a combination of natural and then, if still needed, prescription therapies. The natural therapies recommended here can be dramatically effective in treating anxiety, making you calmer and restoring your peace of mind. They'll also leave you feeling more energetic and mentally clear, instead of drugged out.

Vitamin B$_1$: Taking vitamin B$_1$ decreases anxiety (even panic attacks) and improves mental clarity. Vitamin B$_1$ also helps prevent the production of excess lactic acid, or lactate. Why is this important? A large body of research that was reviewed in the *Journal of Neuropsychiatry and Clinical Neurosciences* in 2001 confirmed that excess sensitivity to high levels of lactic acid is a factor in causing anxiety attacks in people who are prone to them.

The Power of Flower Essences

Bach Flower Remedies, made from a "sun tea" (a sun and boiling method) of wildflowers or trees can work wonders for anxiety. Mimulus can help put fears into perspective, while Aspen flower essence helps to restore a sense of calm and security. A study in the medical journal *Complimentary Health Practice Review* (2007) showed that Bach Rescue Remedy was effective in reducing anxiety. You can use Bach Flower Remedies by adding two drops of the chosen remedy to a glass of water or juice and sipping at intervals or by placing a few drops under the tongue. For more information, visit www.bachremedystore.com.

Vitamin B₃/Niacin: Niacin (vitamin B_3), which is known as a natural tranquilizer, also helps decrease excess lactic acid that can lead to anxiety. You can think of it as "nature's Valium." Niacin has similar effects to Valium on the neurotransmitters that can calm anxiety. More good news: niacin isn't addictive.

Vitamin B₆: Not getting enough vitamin B_6 (pyridoxine) can also contribute to anxiety. That's because you need this vitamin to help you make GABA and serotonin, two of the "happy" brain chemicals that prevent anxiety.

Vitamin B₁₂: You also need vitamin B12 to stay calm. Research done in 1997 by Regland on chronic fatigue syndrome patients has shown that many people require super high levels of B12 to get adequate levels into the brain, where it is needed.

Pantothenic acid: Pantothenic acid is another B vitamin that's critical for the treatment of adrenal fatigue. As we discussed in chapters 2 and 7, adrenal fatigue is a common trigger for hypoglycemia-induced anxiety. If you get irritable when you're hungry, crave sugar, crash with stress, and/or have low blood pressure with dizziness when you stand up, you probably have adrenal fatigue.

Note: You can find all these B vitamins in a good B-complex vitamin.

℞ YOUR WELLNESS PRESCRIPTION

☐ 1. Take 500 mg of vitamin B_1 (thiamine) three times a day.

☐ 2. Take 500+ mcg of vitamin B_{12} a day.

☐ 3. Take one 50+ vitamin B-complex a day.

☐ 4. Take 50 to 100 mg of theanine three times a day.

☐ 5. Take 100 to 200 mg of passionflower extract two or three times a day.

☐ 6. Take one to three capsules of Calming Balance (Health Freedom Nutrition) one to three times a day.

☐ 7. Take 30 mg of magnolia extract three times a day.

☐ 8. Take 200 to 500 mg of magnesium a day.

☐ 9. Use prescription medications as needed.

Theanine: Theanine, which is found in green tea, is a very effective treatment for anxiety. It makes you alert as well as calm. Theanine stimulates the production of alpha brain waves, creating a state of deep relaxation and mental alertness similar to what is achieved through meditation. L-theanine is involved in the formation of the calming neurotransmitter GABA. It also naturally stimulates the release of the "happiness molecules" serotonin and dopamine. For best results, use the natural product SunTheanine, which is the correct natural form needed by the body.

Passionflower extract: A favorite herb for treating anxiety, passionflower was a popular remedy among Native Americans, who first cultivated it. When Spanish conquerors landed in Mexico, they learned about this calming herb from the Aztecs, who used it for insomnia and nervousness. The Spanish brought this plant back to Europe, where it became a go-to remedy to relieve anxiety. Even today, when people in South America are anxious, their friends often tell them to "go get a passionflower drink."

Calming Balance from Health Freedom Nutrition is an outstanding combination supplement for anxiety, and its effect increases with one to four weeks of use. It contains 500 mg of vitamin B1, as well as other B vitamins, passion flower, theanine, magnolia, and magnesium. Check off treatment #10 in appendix A.

Magnolia: Practitioners of Chinese medicine rely on magnolia bark to relieve anxiety without sedating effects. Magnolia extract is chock-full of two phytochemicals: honokiol, which exerts an antianxiety effect, and magnolol, which acts as an antidepressant. This herbal extract relieves stress—even when taken in small doses—and is nonaddictive and nonsedating. You can find these supplements in combination in appendix A. Check off treatment #13 in appendix A.

Magnesium: Magnesium has been called the "antistress mineral" because it relaxes muscles, improves sleep, and relieves tension. Low magnesium levels can trigger hyperventilation, panic attacks, and even seizures if very severe. These attacks can be relieved with magnesium therapy.

It's important to choose the right kind of magnesium. Magnesium oxide and hydroxide are poorly absorbed, but many nutritional supplement manufacturers use this form because it is inexpensive. Choose absorbable forms, such as magnesium citrate or glycinate. Check off treatment #14 in appendix A.

The treatments for types 2 and 4 sugar addiction (see part II), and the natural approaches described above, will effectively resolve anxiety in most people. If severe anxiety persists, consider asking your physician to prescribe a nonaddictive medication called trazodone, which can be helpful—even in very low doses—for treating anxiety. Recommended dose: 25 to 50 mg one to three times a day as needed.

Summary: An Action Plan for Treating Sugar-Related Anxiety

1. Supplement with key nutrients and herbs, such as the B vitamins, magnesium, theanine, passionflower, and magnolia, to calm anxiety naturally.

2. If your anxiety doesn't respond, see your doctor for prescription help.
3. Check off treatments #10, #13, and #14 in appendix A.

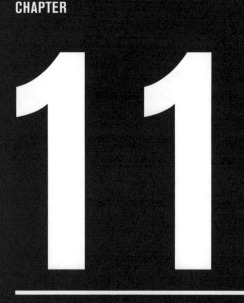

CHRONIC FATIGUE SYNDROME AND FIBROMYALGIA

Do you suffer from persistent, severe fatigue that does not go away with rest? Do you experience horrible insomnia, widespread pain, and severe brain fog? You may have chronic fatigue syndrome (CFS) and/or fibromyalgia (FMS). These two conditions can occur as one type of sugar addiction snowballs into the next, creating a cascade effect. This means you may have symptoms of all four types of sugar addiction simultaneously. More about this in a minute.

CFS and FMS represent an energy crisis. This occurs when you spend more energy than your body is able to make. It's like blowing a fuse. The hypothalamus, which requires an enormous amount of energy, starts to malfunction. This triggers CFS and FMS and can leave you disabled and very ill. The hypothalamus is a major control center in your brain. This center regulates sleep and your hormonal system, body temperature, blood flow, and blood pressure. The good news? The treatment we'll discuss in this section can restore energy production and hypothalamic function, often resulting in full recovery from CFS and FMS.

Inadequate energy levels also result in muscles getting stuck in the shortened position. When this becomes chronic, it causes the myofascial (muscle) pain commonly seen in fibromyalgia. The chronic muscle pain can then cause the pain to generate a pain signal, called central sensitization.

THE CONNECTION BETWEEN SUGAR AND CFS/FMS

CFS/FMS can be triggered in many ways. It can start with a sudden infection or what some experts call "the drop-dead flu." Some folks (who aren't sugar addicts) recover within days to weeks after the infection. However, sugar addicts are much more likely to have yeast overgrowth (type 3 sugar addiction, discussed in chapters 3 and 8), which makes it harder for them to get well. This was the pattern I had when I came down with CFS/FMS in 1975. It knocked me out of medical school and left me homeless for a year before I learned how to recover from these illnesses.

If you are a type 3 sugar addict, when you receive antibiotics for an infection, it flares your yeast overgrowth and may prevent you from recovering. You may then take even more antibiotics for your persistent disabling symptoms (now blamed on the initial infection), which causes you to get worse and worse. Although the initial infection may have triggered your chronic fatigue syndrome, it could also have been aggravated by the antibiotics exacerbating your yeast overgrowth.

In some cases, infections such as the flu can cause direct suppression of the hypothalamus (discussed below), causing adrenal suppression (type 2 sugar addiction, discussed in chapters 2 and 7). When this happens, the result is ever-increasing sugar cravings, which put you on the sugar roller coaster. It also causes suppression of your immune system and yeast overgrowth, so you aren't able to recover without treatment.

Sugar also impairs your immune system. As we mentioned earlier, the amount of sugar in just one can of soda can suppress immune function by 30 percent for three hours. This makes it harder for your body to fight off infections and can enable many kinds of simple infections to turn into chronic fatigue syndrome.

The Snowball Effect: Sugar Addiction and CFS/FMS

Any of the four kinds of sugar addiction can turn into CFS/FMS if untreated, as one type of sugar addiction triggers the next. Over time, carrying the load of all of these different kinds of sugar addiction simply drags the body down and overwhelms it.

First, you may experience a gradual onset of fatigue from overworking. You turn to "loan shark" energy drinks and sodas, full of sugar and caffeine, for an energy boost (type 1 sugar addiction, see chapter 1). The excess sugar intake causes a slowly progressive yeast overgrowth (type 3 sugar addiction, see chapter 3). This yeast overgrowth results in chronic sinusitis and chronic bowel infections (usually misdiagnosed as spastic colon and irritable bowel syndrome). The stress of these chronic infections causes your adrenal glands to become exhausted (type 2 sugar addiction, see chapter 2) and leads to hypothalamic dysfunction. Hypothalamic dysfunction then causes premature reproductive hormone deficiencies (type 4 sugar addiction, see chapter 4). Estrogen deficiency is a major cause of insomnia, and sleep deprivation has been shown to suppress the immune system as well. This can cause more infections, more antibiotics, and more yeast. So the escalating cycle continues.

You can enter this cycle from any of the four types of sugar addiction. The bottom line is, as the cycle progresses, it overwhelms your system and can trigger CFS and FMS.

Having personally treated more than 3,000 patients with CFS and FMS successfully, we have found that sugar addiction is the rule rather than the exception in these illnesses. Beating the sugar addiction is a critical part of the recovery process. But it is only the first step to getting well. We'll show you how to heal your body and feel better than you have ever felt before.

The Growing Problem of Sugar-Related CFS and FMS

As more and more people have grown addicted to sugar and have used it to deal with stress, CFS and FMS have become more common. Over the past decade, CFS and FMS have exploded by 200 to 1,000 percent, as documented in more than eight separate studies in countries throughout Europe and Africa. In the United States, close to 2.5 million people suffer from CFS. Worldwide, the prevalence of FMS has gone up by 200 to 400 percent in the past decade and is now found in 4 to 8 percent of the population. In the United States, this means it affects 12 to 24 million people. The Centers for Disease Control, the National Institutes of Health, and the FDA all now recognize that CFS and FMS are bona fide and devastating illnesses.

THE SHINE PROTOCOL

Although most physicians are simply not trained in recognizing or treating these illnesses, the good news is that CFS and FMS are now very treatable. They do, however, require an "intensive care" approach—treating aggressively with the principles we call the SHINE Protocol. We talked about this in chapter 6; in this chapter, we'll take SHINE to the next level as it relates to people with CFS and FMS.

For instance, type 1 sugar addicts usually will be able to correct their sleep disorders by taking a combination of herbal remedies. However, our research has shown that people with CFS and FMS frequently need three or four different medications, in addition to natural remedies, in order to sleep eight hours a night. Nearly all CFS and FMS patients require treatment for thyroid hormone deficiency, and most require adrenal support and other hormones. Many studies, including a number by Dr. Garth Nicholson, have also shown that a dozen or more infections are present in more than three-quarters of patients with CFS and FMS.

All of this means that treatment for these diseases must be very aggressive and comprehensive in order to restore energy production, eliminate the problems draining your energy, and reset the hypothalamic "circuit breaker" that's been blown. So, in addition to taking the actions prescribed in chapter 6 for type 1 sugar addicts (if you fit the profile in chapter 1), you'll find information in this chapter that is specifically geared to the energy crisis that results in CFS and FMS.

To make this simple, I recommend you do the free "Energy Analysis program" at www.endfatigue.com. It will analyze your symptoms (and even key lab tests if available) to determine exactly which treatments you need. If the following seems a bit complicated, don't worry—the online program will make it easy to determine what you need to do. More about this later. For now, let's look at how you can get well.

Research Shows the SHINE Protocol Works

To effectively treat chronic fatigue syndrome and fibromyalgia, we address five key points we call SHINE:

- Sleep

- Hormonal support

- Infections

- Nutritional support

- Exercise

This is your checklist for recovery. Let's look at the research behind this, and then we'll cover each part of the SHINE treatment.

Research shows that the SHINE Protocol is an effective treatment for CFS and FMS. My groundbreaking study, "Effective Treatment of Chronic Fatigue Syndrome and Fibromyalgia: The Results of a Randomized, Double-Blind, Placebo-Controlled Study," was published in the *Journal of Chronic Fatigue* in 2001, making this effective treatment available to people suffering from these illnesses.

In the study, 91 percent of patients improved with treatment. After three months, the average patient experienced a 75 percent improvement in quality of life. After two years of treatment, the average improvement in quality of life increased to 90 percent—despite patients having been weaned off of most of the treatments. Pain decreased by more than 50 percent on average. Most patients no longer even qualified for the diagnosis of CFS or FMS after treatment. Interestingly, many of the same principles for treating fibromyalgia also apply to myofascial pain syndrome (muscle pain).

The fact that the vast majority of patients improved significantly in the active group while there was minimal improvement in the placebo group proves two important things. The first is that these are very treatable diseases. The second is they are also very real and physical illnesses (otherwise the placebo group would have done as well as those receiving active treatment). The full text of the studies (the study discussed above confirmed an earlier study with the same effect) can be found at www.vitality101.com.

In addition, an editorial published in the April 2002 Journal of the *American Academy of Pain Management*, a major multidisciplinary medical society for pain management in the

United States, noted "the comprehensive and aggressive metabolic approaches to treatment detailed in the Teitelbaum study are all highly successful approaches and make fibromyalgia a very treatment-responsive disorder. The study by Dr. Teitelbaum and others and years of clinical experience make this approach an excellent and powerfully effective part of the standard of practice for treatment of people who suffer from fibromyalgia and myofascial pain syndrome."

Restful Sleep Improves Hypothalmic Function

If you have chronic fatigue syndrome or fibromyalgia, it's very likely that you are unable to get seven to eight hours of deep sleep a night without taking medications. In part, this occurs because hypothalamic function is critical to deep sleep. Your hypothalamic dysfunction requires aggressive sleep support so you can get the healing, deep sleep you need. Unfortunately, many of the most common sleep medications actually aggravate the problem by decreasing the amount of time spent in deep sleep. For patients to get well, they need to take enough of the correct sleep medications to get eight hours of sleep per night. These prescription medications may include Ambien, Desyrel, Neurontin, Klonopin, Lyrica, and, if you don't have Restless Leg Syndrome, Flexeril and/or Elavil. You may also find that over-the-counter antihistamines such as doxylamine (Unisom) or Benadryl can help.

R͓ YOUR WELLNESS PRESCRIPTION

- [ ] 1. Take natural remedies such as theanine, lemon balm, wild lettuce, valerian, passionflower, and hops.

- [ ] 2. Take one to four tablets of 125 mg slow-release magnesium at bedtime.

- [ ] 3. Take 100 to 300 mg of 5-HTP at bedtime.

- [ ] 4. Take 0.5 mg of melatonin at bedtime.

- [ ] 5. Take 25 to 50 mg of over-the-counter antihistamines such as doxylamine or Benadryl (diphenhydramine) at bedtime.

- [ ] 6. Use the correct prescription medications as needed.

Take a combination of these natural and over-the-counter treatments and then (if necessary) add the prescription remedies listed below as needed to get eight hours of sleep a night.

Natural remedies can also help you sleep better—try theanine, lemon balm, wild lettuce, valerian, passionflower, and/or hops. Check off treatment #13 in appendix A. Other natural sleep aids include slow-release magnesium (check off treatment #14), 5-HTP, and melatonin.

During the first six months of treatment, you may sometimes need to take as many as six different sleep treatments simultaneously to get the requisite eight hours of sleep at night. This may seem like a lot of different supplements and medications—especially to people who have medication sensitivity (which is common in people with CFS and FMS). Because of this sensitivity, however, you will do better taking a low dose of several medications than a high dose of one. Treating the sleep disorders in CFS and FMS should be viewed in the same light as treating hypertension. Add one treatment to the next until you get proper control. Use the supplements and medications for as long as they are needed.

After six to eighteen months of feeling well, you can probably dispense with most sleep medications. To offer a margin for safety during periods of stress, it may be wise to continue taking a low dose of a sleep medication or an herbal sleep aid for the rest of your life.

Your doctor may initially be uncomfortable with this approach. But if you realize that CFS/FMS is a physical hypothalamic sleep disorder that won't go away simply by teaching people good sleep hygiene/habits, this approach makes sense. Think of it this way: a doctor wouldn't immediately stop blood pressure or diabetes medicines every time the patient started doing better. Our extensive past experience shows that this approach is safe and essential if you want to get well.

Treating Hormonal Deficiencies Linked with Sugar Addiction

The hypothalamus is the main control center for most of the glands in your body. Because of this, hypothalamic dysfunction causes widespread hormonal deficiencies. It can be very helpful to treat this condition with thyroid, adrenal, ovarian, and/or testicular hormones even if your blood tests are normal. That's because most of the "normal ranges" for our blood tests were not developed in the context of hypothalamic suppression or these syndromes. Also, the normal range for most labs is based on statistical norms (called "2 standard deviations").

This means that out of every 100 people, those with the two highest and lowest scores are considered abnormal and everyone else is defined as normal. According to these guidelines, if you are in between, you don't require treatment. It's like being forced to randomly pick a pair of shoes between the sizes of 5 and 13 (they are all in the "normal range") instead of the size that fits you best.

Bio-identical estrogen and progesterone can help women who have CFS/FMS symptoms that get worse around your period. Bio-identical testosterone can benefit men whose blood tests are in the lowest 25 percent of the normal range (70 percent of men with CFS). Taking low doses of these hormones is fairly safe when used as we discuss earlier and under medical supervision. (You can find information about thyroid hormones in chapter 15, adrenal hormones such as Cortef and DHEA in chapter 7, and ovarian and testicular hormones in chapter 9.)

If you have CFS, fibromyalgia, severe unexplained fatigue or pain (and sometimes even unexplained weight gain with fatigue), it's a good idea to take a therapeutic trial of prescription compounded Thyroid (a mix of T4 and T3). If your doctor won't prescribe it, find a holistic physician, using the "Find a Practioner" page on www.endfatigue.com because these physicians are experts and up-to-date on the research (see appendix C to find a physician).

If you cannot get prescription thyroid, you can also try taking a mixture of thyroid glandulars, plus nutritional and herbal support. You'll find information about a combination formula in appendix A, treatment #15. You'll also learn more about hypothyroidism in chapter 15.

Growth hormone has also been shown to be helpful in treating fibromyalgia. We don't use it often because, unfortunately, it can cost more than $10,000 a year and is given by injection. Fortunately, there are cheaper ways to raise your low growth hormone. Most growth hormone is made during deep sleep, exercise, and sex—I recommend all three!

R̲x YOUR WELLNESS PRESCRIPTION

☐ 1. Take prescription thyroid medication adjusted to the dose that lets you feel best.

☐ 2. Take up to 20 mg of Cortef (hydrocortisone) a day along with natural adrenal support.

☐ 3. Take DHEA if needed, based on your blood tests.

Treating Unusual Infections in Your Sugar-Impaired Immune System

If you have CFS or FMS, it's very likely that your immune system is not functioning the way it should. Excess sugar is a critical immune suppressant. Yeast/candida—fed by the sugar you eat—also contribute to bowel infections, which play a major role in causing CFS/FMS. Not getting enough sleep is another important factor that can cause immune suppression. Nutritional deficiencies (especially zinc) affect immune function, too.

When your immune system is impaired, many unusual infections can take hold. These include viral infections (e.g., HHV-6, CMV, and EBV), parasites and other bowel infections, infections sensitive to long-term treatment with the antibiotics Cipro and Doxycycline (e.g., mycoplasma, chlamydia, Lyme disease, etc.), and fungal infections. Clinical experience shows that treating with prescription antifungals such as Diflucan can help relieve the symptoms seen in these syndromes. (You can learn more about this in the treatment for type 3 sugar addiction in chapter 8.)

Supplementing a Diet of Processed Foods and Sugar

Because the American diet has been highly processed, and 18 percent of our calories come from sugar (devoid of vitamins and minerals), nutritional deficiencies are a common problem. Your body needs more nutrients than normal to heal and fight infections, especially if your immune system is already compromised due to CFS or FMS.

In addition, bowel infections can cause poor nutritional absorption, while your illness itself can cause increased nutritional needs. The most important nutrients you need include B vitamins (especially vitamin B_{12}); the antioxidant vitamins C and E; minerals, especially magnesium, zinc, and selenium; and amino acids.

If you have CFS and FMS, supplementing with a nutrient called ribose can make a huge difference in the amount of energy you have. Ribose is a special, five-carbon sugar that is made naturally in our bodies. But ribose is not like any other sugar.

Sugars we are all familiar with, such as table sugar (sucrose), corn sugar (glucose), milk sugar (lactose), honey (predominantly fructose), and others, are used by the body as fuel. These sugars are consumed and, with the help of the oxygen we breathe, are "burned" by the body to recycle energy. When these sugars are consumed excessively, however, they become toxic, acting as energy loan sharks in the body.

Rx YOUR WELLNESS PRESCRIPTION

- [ ] 1. Take 500+ mcg of vitamin B₁₂ a day.
- [ ] 2. Take 500 to 1,000 mg of vitamin C a day.
- [ ] 3. Take at least 50 mg of B-complex vitamins a day.
- [ ] 4. Take 150 to 500 mg of magnesium a day.
- [ ] 5. Take 15 to 25 mg of zinc a day.
- [ ] 6. Take 150 to 55 mcg of selenium a day.
- [ ] 7. Take 5,000 to 10,000 mg of amino acids a day.
- [ ] 8. Fifty key nutrients (including 1 through 7 above) can be found in vitamin powders. Check off treatment #11 in appendix A.
- [ ] 9. Take 5 grams (5,000 mg) of ribose three times a day for three weeks. You can then drop down to twice a day.

Ribose, on the other hand, is special. It actually has a negative value on the glycemic index. When you consume ribose, your body recognizes that it is different from other sugars and preserves it for the vital work of actually making the special "energy molecules" (ATP, NADH, and FADH) that power your heart, muscles, brain, and every other tissue in your body. Ribose is also critical to the production of DNA and RNA that are the "control centers" in each cell of your body.

A study I published in 2006 in the *Journal of Alternative and Complementary Medicine* shows that patients experienced an average 44.7 percent increase in energy after supplementing with ribose for only three weeks, with improvement beginning at day twelve. They also reported an average of 30 percent overall improvement in quality of life. Two-thirds of the study patients felt they had improved. A new 2012 study done at fifty-seven different treatment centers showed an average 61 percent increase in energy in CFS and fibromyalgia patients taking Ribose!

This latest study published in the *Open Pain Journal* in 2012, showed that using D-ribose resulted in markedly improved energy levels, sleep, mental clarity, pain relief, and well-being in patients suffering from CFS and fibromyalgia. Check off treatment #12 in appendix A.

Get the Latest CFS/FMS Research News

To continue to stay up to date on the cutting edge of CFS/FMS research, sign up for my free e-mail newsletter at www.vitality101.com.

Walk Your Way to Wellness

Start out by walking as much as you can, so that you feel "good tired" afterward and better the next day. Do not push beyond what is comfortable. Otherwise, you're likely to crash and find yourself bed bound the next day. When you reach a comfortable level, stay at that level until you are ten to twelve weeks into the SHINE Protocol treatment. After ten weeks on the program, your energy production will increase. Now you'll be able to increase your walking time by one minute a day, as you feel able.

When you get up to one hour a day, you can increase the intensity of your workout. Add other physical activities, such as swimming, biking, and low-impact aerobics, as long as you feel good about doing it.

℞ YOUR WELLNESS PRESCRIPTION

- [ ] 1. Start a walking program, but only for as many minutes a day as feels good.
- [ ] 2. After ten weeks on the SHINE protocol, increase your walking by up to one minute a day, as you are able.
- [ ] 2. When you are walking one hour a day, you can begin to increase the intensity of your workout by adding other activities.

Dr. T's Online Program to Recover from CFS/FMS

Determining which treatments a patient needs and teaching him or her how to use them can be difficult and time-consuming, even for doctors who are skilled in treating these syndromes. A new patient visit in my office usually takes at least three hours of my one-on-one time. Therefore, I've created a free online program that can help you recover.

Visit my website, www.endfatigue.com, and click on the "Energy Analytics" program for detailed instructions on treatments for each of these problems. The program can analyze your symptoms and, if you have them available, even your lab tests, to tailor a comprehensive individualized treatment protocol to your case using both natural and prescription therapies. It will also tell you which specific problems are causing your CFS/FMS. By showing you how to optimize energy production, it can automatically help you and your holistic physician.

IF YOU STILL HAVE FIBROMYALGIA PAIN AND INFLAMMATION

Your fibromyalgia pain usually will decrease, and often go away, when you follow the SHINE Protocol. But if pain continues to be an issue, avoid medications in the aspirin family (including ibuprofen). They are not very effective for most patients with fibromyalgia and myofascial pain. In addition, the regular use of Tylenol (acetaminophen) can markedly deplete a critical antioxidant (glutathione) in your body. The medications Ultram (tramadol), Skelaxin, Neurontin, Lyrica, Cymbalta, and Savella can be helpful and are safe for fibromyalgia pain. You'll find more treatments for pain in my book: *Pain Free 1-2-3.*

Natural Remedies for Fibromyalgia Pain (and pain in general)

Helpful natural treatments include special extracts of the herbal remedies boswellia serrata, which helps decrease pain and stiffness, white willow bark that contains salicin, an anti-inflammatory compound, and cherry fruit, which has been demonstrated to support healthy uric acid levels. The easiest way to take these herbs is with a combination product called End Pain, which you'll find in appendix A. Check off treatment #15a. This product can be more effective than Celebrex and Motrin and is much safer. Although some effects can be seen immediately, improvement continues to build over a period of six weeks.

My favorite natural product to reduce chronic pain and inflammation is Curamin, from EuroPharma. Curamin is a clinically proven blend of BosPure Boswellia and BCM-95, a very highly absorbable form of curcumin, (turmeric), each with up to ten times the effectiveness of plain or unstandaridized extracts. Check off treatment #15b in appendix A.

The herbal cream, Traumaplant Comfrey Cream (EuroPhama), is also very helpful for relieving pain.

Need Support?

The Fibromyalgia Coalition International (www.fibrocoalition.org) is one of my favorite support groups. Yvonne Keeney is a tireless patient advocate for those suffering fibromyalgia, and their organization has a wide range of resources.

Summary: An Action Plan for Treating CFS and FMS

1. Use the SHINE Protocol to treat your CFS/FMS. SHINE stands for the following:
   S: Sleep
   H: Hormones
   I: Infections
   N: Nutrition
   E: Exercise

2. Complete the free Energy Analysis program at www.endfatigue.com to tailor a comprehensive treatment program to optimize energy in your case.

3. Read my books *The Fatigue and Fibromyalgia Solution* ("an easy read") and *From Fatigued to Fantastic!* ("the textbook"), which will teach you, in detail, how to recover from CFS/FMS.

4. Find a CFS/Fibromyalgia doctor on my website www.endfatigue.com. See the Physician Finder.

5. I treat fatigue, CFS, and fibromyalgia patients from all over the world both in person and by phone consultations and will be happy to help you recover your health and vitality. For more information, see www.vitality101.com, e-mail office@endfatigue.com, and/or call 410-573-5389.

6. Check off treatments #11 to 15, 15a, 15b, and #36 (if you have fibromyalgia pain) in appendix A.

CHAPTER

12

DEPRESSION

Eating sugar can give you the sugar blues. That's because the initial sugar high you get from consuming cookies, candy, soft drinks, etc., quickly wears off and leads to a sugar low that can put you in a downward spiral.

According to the Centers for Disease Control and Prevention (CDC), about 9 percent of adult Americans are depressed. Depression is more than just feeling down or a little blue every now and then. It's a powerful force that can wreak havoc in all aspects of your life, cutting you off from the people you love and sapping the joy from your life.

SUGAR FREE BUT STILL FEEL DOWN?

Even after you've gotten off the sugar roller coaster, you may still experience depression caused by nutritional deficiencies related to excessive sugar intake in the past. In particular, you may need to supplement with fish oil, B vitamins, vitamin D, and magnesium.

Hypothyroidism and low estrogen often accompany sugar addiction and can leave you feeling chronically ill. A low or even low-normal testosterone level is often associated with depression in men. A study in the March 2008 issue of the *Archives of General Psychiatry* shows that older men with abnormally low free testosterone levels are 271 percent more likely to be depressed than those with normal testosterone levels.

Bio-identical testosterone (not to be confused with the dangerous high-dose synthetics that some bodybuilders use) is often more effective than antidepressants for treating depression—even if you have technically "normal" testosterone levels. You can find out more about testosterone in the treatment plan for Type 4 Sugar Addicts on page 127.

These nutritional and hormonal deficiencies, which are common in sugar addicts, can lead to deficiencies in serotonin, dopamine, and norepinephrine (the key mood-regulating chemicals in the brain). This, in turn, can cause you to crave sugar in an attempt to feel better, which feeds the cycle and makes you feel even more depressed.

An underactive thyroid or hypothyroidism is a major cause of depression. (For more information about this, see chapter 15: Hypothyroidism.) Depressed patients who fail on antidepressant medication therapy often respond very well when given thyroid hormone, even though they have normal thyroid blood tests. The catch is that only the active T3 thyroid hormone works for depression. This is not present in the thyroid hormones most physicians prescribe, such as Synthroid (which only contains the inactive T4 thyroid hormone). It is present in prescription "desiccated thyroid glandular" and compounded T3/T4 thyroid combinations.

In 2003, a study done in Israel and published in the *International Journal of Neuropsychopharmacology* followed patients who did not respond to antidepressants—even at a high dose. This group also had severe depression. The active thyroid hormone T3 was added. The thyroid hormone effectively treated the depression in ten of sixteen women patients (62.5 percent), but was not effective in any of the nine male patients who received it. I suspect the men would have found a similar response to optimizing their testosterone levels.

In some cases of severe depression, prescription medicines can be absolutely life saving, but if you are mildly to moderately depressed, you may want to consider other options. Instead of just taking a pill, it can be more effective to look at the underlying causes of your depression, while using natural therapies to support the biochemistry of happiness. When you do this, most depression can be effectively treated—without loss of libido, weight gain, fatigue, or increased risk of suicide that can be the side effects of some prescription antidepressants.

TREATING DEPRESSION WITH NATURAL AND NUTRITIONAL SUPPLEMENTS

When treating depression, it's essential that your body has what it needs to make the three key "happiness" neurotransmitters: serotonin, dopamine, and norepinephrine. B vitamins and magnesium are also critical for energy production, as well as for producing the hormones and neurotransmitters that contribute to feeling good. Other natural remedies like the herbs St. John's wort and magnolia and fish oil can also contribute to happiness. In fact, a study at Harvard Medical School found that among people who have depression or anxiety, more than half use alternative medicine therapies.

Vitamin B$_{12}$ and folic acid: Taking supplements of these two vitamins aids your body's production of both serotonin (the "happiness molecule") and a powerful depression-fighting nutrient called SAMe. Studies of high-dose folic acid have shown this nutrient by itself to be as effective as antidepressant medications, but without unwanted side effects. In a 2005 review in the *Journal of Psychopharmacology*, the authors note, "There is now substantial evidence of a common decrease in folate [and] vitamin B$_{12}$ in depression . . . On the basis of current data, we suggest that oral doses of both folic acid (800 mcg daily) and vitamin B$_{12}$ (1,000 mcg daily) should be tried to improve treatment outcome in depression."

Approximately a third of patients suffering with depression have been found to be deficient in folic acid, and this by itself can cause depression, as can B$_{12}$ deficiency. Taking folic acid and B12 gives your body the building blocks it needs to make you happier.

5-HTP and tyrosine: The same "happiness molecules" raised by prescription antidepressants can be raised naturally—without the side effects. Serotonin is made from 5-HTP. Dopamine and norepinephrine are made from tyrosine. Numerous double-blind studies, including several reported in 1977 in the journal *Archiv für Psychiatrie und Nervenkrankheiten* have shown 5-HTP to be as effective as prescription antidepressants

Rx YOUR WELLNESS PRESCRIPTION

☐ 1. Take 500+ mcg of vitamins B₁₂ and 400 to 800 mcg of folate daily.

☐ 2. Take 50 mg each of vitamin B₂ (riboflavin), B₆ (pyridoxine), and B₃ (niacin) daily. (These can all be found in many "50 mg B-complex" products in a single capsule.)

☐ 3. Take 200 to 500 mg of magnesium a day.

☐ 4. Take 500 to 1,000 mg of tyrosine a day.

☐ 5. Take 200 to 300 mg of 5-HTP a day.

☐ 6. Take 300 to 600 mg of St. John's wort three times a day.

☐ 7. Take 30 mg of magnolia extract three times a day.

☐ 8. Take 1-2 Vectomega fish-oil tablets a day, or eat at least 6 ounces (170 g) of salmon or tuna at least four times a week for three to nine months until the depression clears and then as needed. Check off treatment #16 in appendix A.

☐ 9. Use bio-identical hormones to optimize thyroid and testosterone hormone levels.

☐ 10. Take prescription medications if needed.

☐ 11. Change your attitude—Learn to express your feelings and then let go of them.

☐ 12. Give both natural and prescription antidepressants six weeks to work because it takes this long to fully see their effects. Be aware that suddenly stopping prescription antidepressants can result in severe withdrawal reactions (just like stopping narcotics).

☐ 13. Read the e-book THREE STEPS TO HAPPINESS.

☐ 14. Take CuraMed (750 mg) twice a day. This special Curcumin is as effective as antidepressants.

Seak Releif by Doing Yoga

Researchers at Boston University School of Medicine and McLean Hospital found that practicing yoga may elevate the brain's gamma-aminobutyric (GABA) levels, helping to relieve depression and anxiety. In fact, when people practiced yoga in the study, they felt a similar effect to when they were treated with antidepressants. You can also take GABA as a supplement.

without the adverse side effects. The same goes for tyrosine. Taking tyrosine along with 5-HTP may result in long-lasting improvement. I recommend avoiding doses higher than 200 to 250 mg of 5-HTP if you're on prescription antidepressants to avoid raising serotonin too high. Stop the 5-HTP and discuss with your holistic physician if you get anxiety, racing heart, or fever when combining 5-HTP with prescription antidepressants (or from the antidepressants alone—ask your doctor about serotonergic syndrome).

Riboflavin and niacin: Riboflavin (vitamin B_2) and niacin (vitamin B_3) are key components of the "energy molecules" NADH and FADH, which makes them important players in energy production. If you feel depressed, you may have a niacin and/or riboflavin deficiency.

Vitamin B_6: Depression can also be a result of low vitamin B_6 levels. Vitamin B_6 is critical in the production of serotonin, dopamine, and norepinephrine. A deficiency of B_6 is an especially significant problem in women who take birth control pills or estrogen, both of which can deplete your body's vitamin B_6.

Magnesium: Magnesium deficiency can also contribute to depression, as well as fatigue, pain, and increased risk of heart attack. This mineral is essential for more than 300 different reactions in your body.

St. John's wort: A 2008 review in the highly respected *Cochrane Database of Systematic Reviews* looked at twenty-nine studies involving 5,489 patients with depression and compared treatment with extracts of St. John's wort for four to twelve weeks with placebo treatment or standard antidepressants. The studies mostly included patients suffering from mild to moderately severe symptoms. Overall, the St. John's wort extracts were more effective than a placebo and as or more effective than standard antidepressants.

Magnolia: Practitioners of Chinese medicine have long relied on magnolia bark to treat depression. Magnolia extract is rich in two phytochemicals: honokiol, which eases anxiety, and magnolol, which acts as an antidepressant. It is a nonaddictive, nonsedating antidepressant. For a combination product that contains all of these nutrients and herbals, check off treatment #17 in appendix A.

Curcumin (CuraMed): Two new studies showed this special, highly absorbed curcumin is as effective as prescription antidepressants after six weeks. It was shown to be even more effective for severe depression. Take 750 mg twice a day. It must be the CuraMed form, however, as others require more than 16 capsules a day.

Fish Oil: The brain is 60 percent fat, and if you aren't getting enough of Omega 3 fatty acids that enable neurons to communicate with each other, this can lead to depression. The Eicosapentaenoic acid (EPA) found in fish oils can even improve the effectiveness of anti-depressant medications. Just choose a high quality brand that is free from toxins. I recommend Vectromega (EuroPharma) in which 1–2 tablets replace 8–16 fish oil capsules.

Prescription antidepressants: If your depression is severe, or when natural therapies are not effective, prescription antidepressants such as Prozac, Paxil, and Wellbutrin can help by raising levels of the neurotransmitters serotonin, dopamine, and norepinephrine in

More Natural Depression Treatments

- Research shows that acupuncture is a promising treatment for depression in women. A study at the University of Arizona with thirty eight women with mild to moderate depression showed that after twelve sessions, 70 percent of women experienced at least a 50 percent reduction of symptoms, results comparable to the success rate of psycho-therapy and medication.

- Bach Flower Remedies are made from a 'sun tea' of specific wildflowers or trees known for their healing properties and then diluted (similar to homeopathic remedies in that regard). The Star of Bethlehem, Gorse, Crap Apple, Elm, and Wild Rose can all help improve optimism. Visit http://www.bachcentre.com/centre/remedies.htm to see which is right for you.

Use Caution Combining Remedies

If you are combining St. John's wort with prescription antidepressants, it is best to use lower doses (300 mg three times a day) under the guidance of a holistic health practitioner. The combination of these two remedies can drive serotonin levels too high, resulting in serotonergic syndrome. This can lead to anxiety, rapid pulse, and, when severe, even fever. In rare instances, it can even be life threatening. The same problem can occur with 5-HTP. If symptoms occur while you are on antidepressants, stop taking St. John's wort and 5-HTP and let your holistic physician know. Also consult your physician immediately about lowering the medication dose. Don't stop the medication suddenly because it could result in severe withdrawal symptoms.

your body. Unfortunately, these medications can sometimes be toxic and produce unwanted side effects. It's best to discuss with your doctor what is right for you.

Note: Do not try to "tough it out" if you are severely depressed. Get the help you need from a therapist and/or a health care practitioner. Also the e-book *Three Steps to Happiness* can be dramatically helpful, as well. Follow the simple directions and you'll feel much better.

THE LINK BETWEEN DEPRESSION AND ANGER

From a psychological perspective, depression usually represents anger that has been repressed or turned inward. If you're depressed, allowing yourself to be angry can be healthy. You can tell when the anger is healthy because it will feel good. Remember, though, that you are choosing to be angry, and what you are angry about is nobody else's fault. Violence is not a healthy or an acceptable expression of anger.

You may notice that you feel better after you allow yourself to express and release your anger, and your depression may decrease. Sometimes, a session with a therapist can be a safe place to do this. If you have persistent depression that does not respond to treatment, see a professional.

Change Your Attitude to Ease Depression

1. Feel all of your feelings without the need to understand or justify them. When they no longer feel good, let go of them.

2. Make life a "no-fault" system. This means *no blame, no fault, no guilt, no judgment, and no expectations* toward yourself or anyone else. If you find yourself judging somebody, simply stop yourself as soon as you notice it. And no judging yourself for judging others.

3. Learn to keep your attention focused on what feels good. We sometimes are given the misconception that paying attention to our problems is more realistic. Not so. Life is like a massive buffet with thousands of options. You can choose where you want to put your attention—put it on things that feel good. If a problem truly requires your attention, it will feel good to focus on it and handle it. Otherwise, it's like filling your plate at that buffet with only things you don't like.

4. Look on the bright side. According to the *Mayo Clinic Health Letter* in 2009, cultivating a positive outlook can improve health and decrease the risk of depression. You're also likely to live longer. Their data comes from research conducted in the Women's Health Initiative, a study of almost 100,000 women aged fifty and older.

5. Keep a daily gratitude list. It's a good way to get into the habit of seeing the glass half-full instead of half-empty. Every morning, write down five things you are grateful for. When you find yourself going to the dark side during the day, remind yourself of these five things and you'll feel more optimistic.

Summary: An Action Plan for Treating Depression

1. Treat your depression naturally with B vitamins, magnesium, tyrosine, 5-HTP, St. John's wort, magnolia extract, and fish oil.

2. Use bio-identical hormones as needed.

3. If your depression is severe, see a health practitioner for a prescription medication.

4. Learn to express anger in a healthy way and then focus on the positive.

5. Check off #16 and #17 in appendix A.

6. Read the E-book *Three Steps to Happiness*.

13

DIABETES AND METABOLIC SYNDROME

Diabetes is an illness found almost exclusively in countries and societies where there is an overconsumption of sugar. Type 1 diabetes (occurring mostly in children) is associated with destruction of the cells in the pancreas, which makes insulin. Adult-onset diabetes (type 2) is usually associated with very high levels of insulin in the blood. Unfortunately, the insulin does not work (this is called insulin resistance). In either type, a lack of insulin or insulin effectiveness makes it hard for sugar to move out of your blood vessels and into your cells, where it would be burned as fuel. This results in excessive and toxic sugar levels in the blood, which can lead to heart attacks, strokes, nerve pain, and multiple other severe medical conditions.

Because sugar is the key factor in causing and driving the illness, diabetes—particularly type 2 diabetes—can be a problem for many sugar addicts. Drinking just one 12-ounce (355 ml) sugar-sweetened soft drink a day can increase the risk of type 2 diabetes by 22 percent, according to a 2013 study from the School of Public Health, Imperial College London, United Kingdom, and published online in *Diabetologia*.

A study published in the *Archives of Internal Medicine* in 2008 shows in detail just how sugary drinks impact health. Researchers studied 43,960 African-American women and found that the incidence of type 2 diabetes was higher in women who had a greater intake of both sugar-sweetened soft drinks and fruit drinks. Drinking at least two soft drinks per day was associated with a 24 percent increased risk of type 2 diabetes, and consumption of at least two fruit drinks per day was associated with a 31 percent increase. Epidemiologic studies show that diabetes is almost unheard of in black populations in Africa—until a Western diet high in sugar and low in fiber is introduced. Then diabetes rates skyrocket. The same problem was seen in Native American populations in the United States.

Ideally, your body makes insulin to carry sugar from the blood into your cells, where it can be burned as fuel. But in type 1 diabetes, the cells that manufacture insulin have been destroyed, so you just don't have the cells you need to make insulin so that you can process sugar.

In type 2 diabetes (the condition we discuss here as it relates to sugar addiction), your body gets overwhelmed by the demands of processing excess sugar. Eating sugar can also make you overweight, a key risk factor for type 2 diabetes. When you are a type 2 diabetic, you manufacture plenty of insulin, but it just doesn't work. This is what's known as "insulin resistance." Unfortunately, a high insulin level makes you continue to pack on pounds of body fat, which then worsens the insulin resistance.

If you are a type 1 (childhood) diabetic, it's important to follow the recommendations of your doctor. Several natural remedies can help as well. We'll note those as we go along. But in this section, our main focus is type 2 (adult-onset) diabetes and metabolic syndrome. Metabolic syndrome means you have insulin resistance along with high blood pressure, weight gain, elevated cholesterol, and often diabetes, which increases your risk of heart attack if not treated.

Do you have metabolic syndrome? You must have three of these five risk factors:

1. A large waistline

2. High blood pressure

3. High triglycerides

4. Low levels of "good" HDL cholesterol

5. Diabetes/high blood sugar (associated with insulin resistance)

In men, metabolic syndrome is often caused by testosterone deficiency (a blood level under 450 should be treated). Testosterone plays an important role in glucose metabolism, and for this reason, low testosterone can be a major factor in the development of diabetes and metabolic syndrome. In addition, large epidemiologic studies have shown a strong association between type 2 diabetes and low testosterone levels. For example, in the Third National Health and Nutrition Examination Survey (NHANES III) that looked at more than 1,400 men, those men whose free testosterone levels were in the lowest third of the population were four times more likely to have diabetes than men in the highest third.

Interestingly, in addition to low testosterone causing diabetes in men, the converse is true. Diabetes can probably lower testosterone as well. A 2008 study published in *Diabetes Care* found that about a third of men between the ages of eighteen and thirty-five who have type 2 diabetes also have low testosterone (because the hypothalamic/pituitary hormonal control center in the brain is not stimulating the testes).

The potential implications for men, in terms of their sexual and reproductive function during prime reproductive years, are "profound," notes Dr. Paresh Dandona and colleagues from the State University of New York at Buffalo.

Fortunately, a low testosterone level can usually be treated using safe, bio-identical, natural testosterone. (You can learn more about bio-identical testosterone hormone treatment in chapter 9.)

In addition, if you have metabolic syndrome and high hostility levels, you have a fourfold risk of having a heart attack compared to people without these cardiovascular risk factors, according to a study by researchers at Brown University, published in the July 2005 issue of the *American Journal of Cardiology*.

On the plus side, research published in the medical journal *Andrologia* in 2008 showed that testosterone therapy can improve metabolic syndrome in men, decreasing the risk of diabetes and heart disease. You can find out more about heart disease later in this section.

In women, paradoxically, an elevated testosterone level can cause diabetes. This is seen in women who have polycystic ovarian syndrome (PCOS) and have high testosterone levels and insulin resistance. The information in this book can help PCOS as well, including avoiding sugar, optimizing the correct types of estrogen, and treating adrenal exhaustion. (See chapter 7.)

TREATING TYPE 2 DIABETES

The first step in the treatment of type 2 diabetes is eliminating sugar from your diet. But more is needed to control this illness and its complications. Following this wellness prescription will help restore your body's own insulin sensitivity and often will make type 2 diabetes go away. In addition, it will often help prevent and reverse many of the complications of diabetes.

Lose Weight to Decrease Insulin Resistance

To treat type 2 diabetes (or prevent it), it's important to lose weight if you are overweight. Exercising enough to maintain a healthy body weight decreases insulin resistance and is often enough to make the diabetes go away. A study published in the *American Journal of Cardiology* in 2007 shows the benefits of walking thirty minutes a day six days a week. Researchers found that just taking this action is enough to lose weight and cut the risk of metabolic syndrome (a key cause of heart attack and stroke) by 25 percent—without changing your diet.

Before participants in the STRRIDE study (Studies of a Targeted Risk Reduction Intervention through Defined Exercise) exercised regularly, 41 percent of the study subjects (171 middle-aged, overweight men and women) met the criteria for metabolic syndrome. At the end of the eight-month exercise program, only 27 percent did.

Another benefit of walking? By walking outdoors, you'll increase your sun exposure, which enables your body to manufacture vitamin D. This decreases the risk of diabetes, hypertension, and cancer (vitamin D deficiency is responsible for more than 85,000 cancer deaths a year in the United States).

℞ YOUR WELLNESS PRESCRIPTION

Recommendations 1, 2, and 3 below apply to both type 1 and type 2 diabetics. Recommendations 4 to 7 are only for type 2 adult diabetics.

☐ 1. Eliminate sugar intake and lose weight if you are overweight.

☐ 2. Optimize nutritional support.

☐ a. Increase your fiber intake. Aim for 25 to 50 grams a day. Eat fruits and vegetables that score low on the glycemic index. (See appendix B.)

☐ b. Take vitamin C (500 mg) and vitamin E (100 IU) daily.

☐ c. Take vitamins B_{12} (500 mcg), B_6 (25 to 100 mg), and inositol (500 to 1,000 mg) daily.

☐ d. Take 1,000 to 2,000 IU of vitamin D a day.

☐ e. Take 200 mg of magnesium a day.

☐ 3. Take special nutrients to prevent and treat diabetic nerve injury.

☐ a. Take 1,000 to 2,000 mg of acetyl-L-carnitine a day.

☐ b. Take 300 mg of alpha-lipoic acid twice a day.

☐ 4. Take 200 mg of coenzyme Q10 daily, if you are on cholesterol-lowering medications.

☐ 5. Eat salmon or tuna at least three or four times a week and/or supplement with one Vectomega fish oil tablet.

☐ 6. For men with a blood testosterone level under 450, consider bio-identical testosterone hormone by prescription.

☐ 7. Take Metformin (along with vitamin B_{12}).

Research published in the *American Journal of Clinical Nutrition* in 2004 showed that people with low levels of vitamin D had almost three times the risk of metabolic syndrome. Vitamin D levels also tend to be low in diabetic children. A study published in *Hormone and Metabolic Research* in 2005 showed that vitamin D, when given early, may even help prevent diabetes. The research also shows that the **risk for type 1 diabetes decreased 78 percent** in subjects who took 2,000 IU a day of vitamin D.

The Role of Diet in Treating Diabetes

What you eat plays a key role in type 2 diabetes. In addition to avoiding excess sugar and white flour, you'll want to increase the amount of fiber you eat, along with fruits and vegetables that score low on the glycemic index. (You'll find a glycemic index chart of various foods in appendix B.)

A review of several studies (called a meta-analysis), which was published in the *Journal of the American College of Nutrition*, found that optimizing fiber, carbohydrate, and protein intakes resulted in lower blood sugar levels, as well as improvements in cholesterol and other blood fats. The study recommended that diabetics get 55 percent of their calories from complex carbohydrates and 12 to 16 percent from protein.

Oils should be predominantly liquid unsaturated fats, such as fish oils and olive oil. Dietary fiber should be 25 to 50 grams per day. Overall, instead of counting calories and trying to figure out what percent of your diet should come from what (the numbers above are meant to simply give you a rough idea), find a healthy diet that feels comfortable to you and that you can live with happily. The key points are to avoid sugar, eat relatively unprocessed high-fiber foods that score below 55 on the glycemic index, and use liquid oils.

The Value of Antioxidants

Research shows that the antioxidants we get from food, such as vitamin C, can also lower the risk of diabetes. In a study published in the *Archives of Internal Medicine* in 2008, participants who ate the most fruit and vegetables were found to have a 22 percent lower risk of developing diabetes.

You can also up your antioxidant quotient by taking a good vitamin powder that contains vitamin C and other key nutrients. Supplementing with vitamins and minerals is very important for diabetics because as excess sugar washes out into the urine, it can drag along many other nutrients and wash them out of the body, too. This can lead to widespread nutritional deficiencies, one of the most common is magnesium.

A review of seven studies published in the *Journal of Internal Medicine* in 2007 analyzed data from 286,668 participants and 10,912 people who later developed diabetes. The overall risk of developing diabetes was decreased by 14 percent for each 100 mg/day increase in their daily magnesium intake. You can also add magnesium to your diet by eating more nuts, beans, whole grains, and green leafy vegetables. If you are a diabetic with kidney failure, you'll need your doctor's supervision before supplementing with magnesium.

Nerve-Protecting Nutrients: Acetyl-L-Carnitine, Alpha-Lipoic Acid, and Coenzyme Q10

Acetyl-L-carnitine (ALC) can help ease diabetic neuropathy. Research published online in the *Annals of Pharmacotherapy* in 2008 showed that supplementing with 2,000 mg daily of ALC helped ease diabetic nerve pain significantly. Take it with 300 mg of alpha-lipoic acid twice a day for best results. You can expect to see improvement in about six weeks, though it may take twelve months to gain the full benefit. (Check off treatments #18 and #19 in appendix A.)

Taking cholesterol-lowering medications called "statins" can deplete coenzyme Q10 (CoQ10), causing deficiency. This can cause weakening of the heart muscle and may aggravate diabetic nerve injury, so if you are taking cholesterol medication, also take 200 mg a day of chewable coenzyme Q10. Check off treatment #21 in appendix A.

Supplementation with coenzyme Q10 can also benefit metabolic syndrome. Research published in the *Journal of Pharmacology Sciences* in 2008 showed that CoQ10 reduced oxidative stress and inflammation and improved blood vessel health. This is important because these two factors figure into metabolic syndrome and the heart disease that can result.

Fish Oil

Fish oil decreases inflammation and can protect a diabetic's heart while also normalizing high levels of blood fats called triglycerides. Fish oil is also important for the prevention of type 1 diabetes.

Between 1994 and 2006, scientists in Colorado followed the diet of 1,770 young children at high risk of developing type I diabetes. They found that a high dietary intake of omega-3 fatty acids, found in fish oils, lowered the children's chances of developing diabetes by around 55 percent. In one study, risk of type 1 diabetes decreased by 19 percent when cod liver oil was taken four or fewer times per week and by 26 percent when cod liver oil was given more than five times per week. Risk for type 1 diabetes was lower if cod liver oil was started when the infants were between seven and twelve months old rather than between birth and six months of age. Fish oil may also be heart protective in diabetics. Eat 3 to 4 servings of tuna or salmon a week or take fish oil.

Low Testosterone Can Cause Diabetes

Low testosterone in men can cause diabetes. Insulin resistance can be improved by optimizing testosterone levels using bio-identical hormones. (See chapter 9.)

Metformin: An Excellent Diabetic Medicine

Metformin may be the best diabetic medication to protect your heart. A major review of forty studies, published in the *Archives of Internal Medicine* in 2008, showed that Metformin reduced cardiovascular risk by 26 percent. Rosiglitazone (Avandia), another more expensive antidiabetic medication, actually showed a possible higher risk of heart disease.

Holistic doctors have used Metformin, an excellent, old, and inexpensive medication, for years to treat diabetes and insulin resistance. It can also help you lose weight when insulin resistance is present. Metformin can cause vitamin B_{12} deficiency, so be sure to take vitamin B_{12} with it.

Summary: An Action Plan for Treating Diabetes

1. Supplement with nutrients, including vitamin C, vitamin B_{12}, inositol, vitamin D, CoQ10, acetyl-L-carnitine, alpha-lipoic acid, magnesium, and fish oil.

2. Eat more fiber and fruits and vegetables with low glycemic index scores.

3. Consider bio-identical hormone treatment.

4. Check off treatments #18, #19, and #21, (if needed) in appendix A.

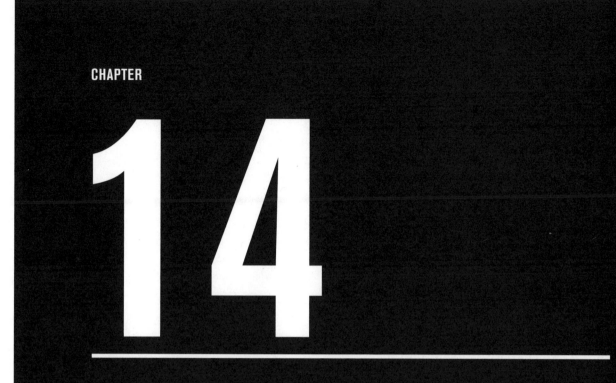

CHAPTER

14

HEART DISEASE

Heart disease was extremely rare a century ago, before we increased our sugar consumption. Today, our high sugar intake can trigger insulin resistance and diabetes, as well as magnesium deficiency, which all have an impact on heart health. Heart diseases that are more common among people with a high sugar intake include angina and heart attacks (the single biggest killer in the United States), congestive heart failure, and even abnormal heart rhythms (arrhythmias). With congestive heart failure, the heart muscle is weakening. With angina, there may not be heart muscle weakness until after a heart attack occurs.

The High Cost of Too Much Sugar

A study in *JAMA Internal Medicine* (2014), an analysis of 25 years of data, revealed that American adults consume on average about 15 percent of their calories from sugars added to foods during processing, with a whopping 37 percent of the added sugar consumed in sugar-sweetened beverages. Researchers projected that drinking just one 12-ounce (355 ml) sugary soda a day may increase the risk of cardiovascular disease by about 30 percent—independent of total calories, obesity, or other risk factors.

TREATING AND PREVENTING HEART DISEASE

By increasing heart efficiency, you can decrease its work and therefore decrease the tendency toward chest pain and abnormal heart rhythms as well. Obviously, cutting back on sugar is an important part of prevention (and preventing further damage). However, there are several very effective and promising natural treatments that can help decrease symptoms and improve the ability to function (e.g., walking, working, and generally living life) in people with heart disease. These natural remedies are safe and inexpensive and usually produce results in six weeks.

Boost Energy with the "Special" Sugar Ribose

Ribose is a five-carbon "special" sugar found in our bodies. Unlike table sugar, corn sugar, or milk sugar, which can be toxic when consumed, ribose is a building block for the energy molecules ATP, FADH, NADH, and acetyl-CoA, which are essential as the energy currency of the cell. ATP powers your heart, muscles, brain, and every other tissue in your body.

But when the heart doesn't have enough energy, it doesn't relax between beats. This means it can't fill completely with blood. Because of this, the heart can't function properly and pump enough blood to the body. When this happens, your tissues become oxygen starved. Ultimately, a heart attack can result or you may experience symptoms of heart failure such as ankle swelling or shortness of breath while exercising or lying flat.

☐ 1. Take one scoop (5 grams) of ribose (Corvalen) three times a day for six weeks, then twice a day thereafter.

☐ 2. Take 400 mg of coenzyme Q10 a day for six weeks, then 200 mg a day thereafter.

☐ 3. Take 200 mg of magnesium a day (only with your doctor's OK if you have kidney failure).

☐ 4. Take 50+ mg of B-complex per day.

☐ 5. Take 500 mg of acetyl-L-carnitine twice a day for six to twelve weeks and then 500 mg per day. (It can often simply be stopped after three to six months.)

☐ 6. Eat two 6-ounce (170 g) servings of oily fish per week or one tablet of Vectromega each day. If you have had a heart attack, eat seven or more servings a week or take two Vectromega fish oil tablets each day.

☐ 7. Take 200 mg of hawthorn extract three times a day if you have heart failure.

☐ 8. Take magnesium orotate 6000 mg a day for one month and then 3000 mg a day (only with your doctors ok if you have kidney failure).

Research shows that ribose has a profound effect on heart function in patients with heart disease. One study published in the *European Journal of Heart Failure* in 2003 showed that when patients with congestive heart failure took 10 grams of ribose daily their heart function increased significantly. Give it six weeks to see the effect. I recommend 5 grams three times a day for the first six weeks. (A brand called Corvalen has a handy

5-gram scoop in the container.) Supplementing with ribose gives the heart the energy it needs to relax, fill with blood, and pump powerfully and easily. This means blood (and the oxygen it contains) is able to circulate the way it is supposed to, and the heart functions far more efficiently—reducing chest pain and shortness of breath and improving stamina. Check off treatment #20 in appendix A.

Take Coenzyme Q10 to Improve Heart Function

This nutrient is critical for energy production and, in turn, for the heart. A review of more than a dozen studies published in both the *Annual of Pharmacotherapy* (2005) and the *Journal of Cardiac Failure* (2006) showed that coenzyme Q10 (CoQ10) increases heart function significantly in heart failure patients.

CoQ10 is especially important if you are on cholesterol-lowering medications, even if you don't have a heart problem, because these medications cause coenzyme Q10 deficiency. This can lead to or aggravate congestive heart failure, and your physician may have no idea that the cholesterol medicine might be contributing to the problem. Coenzyme Q10 levels are also sometimes lower if you use oral contraceptives or Premarin or Provera, which may in turn increase your risk of cardiovascular disease. Check off treatment #21 in appendix A.

Take Magnesium to Strengthen Your Heart

Magnesium deficiency not only decreases your heart muscle's strength but also markedly decreases the tendency of normal heart rhythms. Almost all Western diets are low in magnesium because our food loses more than half of its magnesium through processing. If your magnesium supplement causes diarrhea, use a sustained-release form of magnesium (e.g., Jigsaw Health Sustained-Release Magnesium, which can be taken at bedtime as well to improve sleep). Check off treatment #4 in appendix A.

If you have congestive heart failure, add a special form of magnesium called magnesium orotate. Take 6,000 mg a day for one month, then 3,000 mg a day thereafter. In a placebo-controlled study published in the *International Journal of Cardiology* in 2009, this simple and cheap treatment decreased the death rate in patients with severe congestive heart failure by a whopping 50 percent and improved heart function dramatically as well. It can be easily found online. Check off treatment #22 in appendix A. Keep in mind if you have kidney problems you can only take magnesium if approved by your physician.

Vitamin B-Complex Helps Prevent Heart Failure

B-complex vitamins are also a critical part of the energy molecules (e.g., FADH and NADH) made by your body. Suboptimal levels of these B vitamins play a role in heart failure.

The Importance of Antioxidants, Zinc, Copper, and Iron in Heart Health

Research indicates the importance of antioxidants in preventing heart disease. The minerals zinc, copper, and iron are also important for heart health. A study published in the medical journal *Angiology* in 2008 showed that if you have optimal antioxidant levels, your heart stents are less likely to get blocked up. A study published in *Clinica Chimica Acta* in 2008 suggested that high iron and copper levels and low zinc levels are associated with an increased risk of heart attacks. That's because iron and copper are oxidative (i.e., the opposite of antioxidants).

Take Acetyl-L-Carnitine to Lose Weight

Carnitine is important for many functions in the body, one of which is helping mitochondria produce energy. It you don't have enough carnitine, the body has a tough time burning fat, and this can make you pile on the pounds. You'll find L-carnitine in meat (the word *carni-vore* comes from the carnitine in meat). But it's important to choose the right kind of carnitine. It must be acetyl-L-carnitine; otherwise, it has trouble getting into the mitochondrial "energy furnaces" in your cells, where it works to burn off calories. It also improves heart function. Check off treatment #19 in appendix A.

Take Fish Oil to Prevent Heart Disease

In 2008, the American Heart Association (AHA) endorsed the use of omega-3 fatty acids to help prevent heart disease, especially in people who have coronary artery disease (CAD). Fish oil may also decrease the risk of abnormal heart rhythms and sudden cardiac death.

A study published in the *International Journal of Cardiology* in 2008 showed that long-term fish consumption can even lower the risk of having another heart attack. When the study's participants—214 men and 79 women who had previously had heart attacks—consumed seven or more portions of fish a week, they had a much lower risk of having another heart attack in the next thirty days. Eighty-three percent reduced their risk of recurrent heart problems after hospitalization. If you prefer, take a single tablet of Vectomega daily, which replaces 8–16 fish oil capsules.

Many large studies, totaling more than 300,000 people, confirm the beneficial aspects of omega-3 fatty acid intake. The group that supplemented with omega-3 fatty acids had a 19 to 45 percent reduction in heart attacks. Cholesterol-lowering medications only decrease heart attack deaths by 1.4 percent.

The 2007 large-scale clinical trial conducted by Dr. Yokoyama and colleagues, called the Japan EPA Lipid Intervention Study (JELIS), included more than 18,000 men and women. Almost 15,000 participants had no record of coronary artery disease (primary prevention). Results showed a 19 percent decrease in major coronary events (fatal plus nonfatal) for all subjects, a 19 percent decrease for secondary prevention subjects, and an 18 percent decrease for primary prevention subjects. This effect was still lower than some other studies because the Japanese population already eats a lot of fish.

The large, well-conducted secondary prevention trial, GISSI, included more than 10,000 men. It found a 15 percent decrease in all deaths plus nonfatal heart attacks and strokes, a 26 percent decrease in cardiovascular deaths plus nonfatal heart attacks and strokes, and a 45 percent decrease in sudden death among people taking 1,000 mg a day of fish oil concentrate.

The American Heart Association's recommendation is to eat two meals of oily fish per week (mackerel, herring, tuna, or salmon) to obtain the omega-3 fatty acids needed. However, supplementation with a good-quality fish oil is also beneficial. Check off treatment #23 in appendix A.

Hawthorn Extract Decreases Heart Failure Symptoms

A recent major medical review of fourteen placebo-controlled studies (see *Cochrane Database Systematic Reviews*, 2008) involving more than 1,000 patients found the herb hawthorn to be helpful in treating the symptoms of heart failure. In the review, hawthorn extract was shown to significantly decrease symptoms and improve exercise performance in patients with chronic heart failure—without significant unwanted side effects. Hawthorn extract strengthened heart muscle contraction while increasing blood flow to the heart muscle. This makes it a good remedy for heart failure (which causes shortness of breath during exertion, swollen ankles, and shortness of breath while lying flat). The data suggest hawthorn extract may also be helpful for angina. Recommended dose: 400 mg three times a day.

Alpha-Linolenic Acid Helps Prevent a Second Heart Attack

Tofu and other forms of soybeans and canola, walnut, flaxseed, and their oils all contain alpha-linolenic acid, which can become omega-3 fatty acids in the body. Their benefits to the heart are more modest than what fish oils provide, but a 2008 study published in the journal *Circulation* showed that people who'd already had a heart attack reduced their risk of another by consuming vegetable oils that contain alpha-linolenic acid.

Study subjects whose consumption of these vegetable oils was in the highest 20 percent of the group had a 59 percent lower risk of heart attack than those whose consumption was in the lowest 20 percent. You can also take an alpha-linolenic acid supplement.

Supplement with Bio-identical Testosterone to Protect Your Heart

More and more studies are showing that low testosterone in men is associated with increased death at a younger age, especially from heart disease. A study published in the *Journal of Endocrinology and Metabolism* in 2008, which involved 794 men fifty to ninety-one years of age in the Rancho Bernardo area of California, showed that men with the lowest testosterone levels were more likely to die of heart disease than those with higher levels of testosterone. Treatment with bio-identical testosterone hormones can aid this deficiency and help prevent death from coronary disease. (See chapter 9 for more information.) Fifty milligrams of the topical cream is usually enough. Starting with too high a dose (e.g., 100 mg per day) is like exercise; it does not cause heart disease, but too much can unmask undiagnosed heart disease.

Summary: An Action Plan for Treating Heart Disease

1. Take ribose, coenzyme Q10, and acetyl-L-carnitine to strengthen your heart by boosting overall energy production. Allow six weeks to see the benefits.

2. Get good overall nutritional support in a vitamin powder containing 50 mg of B-complex, 150 to 200 mg of magnesium glycinate, 500 to 750 mg of vitamin C, 100 IU of vitamin E, 15 mg of zinc, 0.5 mg of copper, and other antioxidants. (See appendix A, treatment #1 for a recommended vitamin powder that combines all of these.)

3. Take fish oil tablets (Vectomega) or eat at least 4 ounces (115 g) of fish (salmon, tuna, sardines, herring, or mackerel) three or four times a week—to protect your heart.

4. Take hawthorn extract and magnesium orotate, along with the nutrients above if you have heart failure. Allow six weeks for them to work.

5. Stay on the regimen for a total of three months to see the optimal effects of the regimen. Then you can lower the doses and cut back on the supplements as able.

6. Work with a holistic physician to optimize testosterone levels (in men) and thyroid levels (in women).

7. Check off treatments #4 (as needed), #19, #20, #21, #22, and #23 in appendix A.

15

THYROIDISM

ave hypothyroidism, chances are good that you reach for sugar to get the energy you
function. Severe fatigue is a hallmark of hypothyroidism, often accompanied by
s, brain fog, confusion, constipation, depression, weight gain, intolerance to cold,
skin. Untreated, hypothyroidism can even lead to elevated cholesterol, heart disease,
iages, and infertility. But it's the fatigue that will drive your sugar addiction and put you
wnward spiral. Now that you're off sugar, it's time to treat your hypothyroidism, and get
rgy you need in a healthy way.

ortunately, most people who need thyroid hormone will have normal blood tests, so your
may say you're fine when you're not. More about this in a minute. The good news is that
reating with prescription desiccated (natural) thyroid hormones, or better yet a
nded T4/T3 prescription thyroid hormone, can dramatically improve how you feel.

ou do not get treatment for your hypothyroidism, the fatigue you experience will *not* go
aving you craving sugar in an attempt to get an energy boost. Not treating your low
usually results in unnecessary weight gain as well. This can then trigger the sleep
and fatigue discussed in chapter 1, which can drive sugar cravings.

THE THYROID GLAND'S JOB

The thyroid is a butterfly-shaped gland at the base of your neck. Think of it as the "master of your metabolism." When it's working the way it should, you feel good and have the energy you need to "meet life." When it isn't, you can feel miserable, without understanding why.

Hashimoto's thyroiditis is the most common cause of hypothyroidism. What this means in simplest terms is that antibodies (your body's own immune system) are attacking your thyroid, and will eventually destroy it. This can be diagnosed by a blood test called an anti-TPO antibody. If test results show you have elevated levels of these antibodies, you probably have Hashimoto's thyroiditis.

The thyroid makes two primary hormones. Thyroxin (T4) is the storage form of thyroid hormone. The body uses it to make triiodothyronine (T3), the active form of thyroid hormone.

Most synthetic thyroid medications, such as Synthroid and Levothroid, are pure T4. These synthetics are fine if your body has the ability to properly turn them into triiodothyronine (T3). But not everyone does. For these people, a natural compounded thyroid hormone containing both T4 and T3—or supplementing the Synthroid with Cytomel (T3 thyroid hormone)—can help. You'll learn about this later on in this chapter.

THE PROBLEM WITH LAB TESTS FOR HYPOTHYROIDISM

Most doctors still rely on what is known as the TSH, or thyroid stimulating test, to determine whether you have hypothyroidism. TSH is the molecule made by your brain that is controlled by the hypothalamus/pituitary centers and tells your thyroid how much hormone to make. If TSH is high (i.e., your brain is saying to make more thyroid), a doctor will presume that your thyroid level is low. A high TSH equals low thyroid in medical care. Unfortunately, this test is unreliable and misses millions of folks who need to be treated.

Let's look at the problem with lab testing a bit further. The normal range for thyroid hormone levels is based on statistical norms (called two standard deviations). This means that out of every one hundred people, those with the two highest and lowest scores are considered abnormal—everyone else is defined as normal.

In 2002, the American Academy of Clinical Endocrinologists (AACE), the nation's largest organization of thyroid specialists, recommended that doctors consider treatment for patients who have a TSH level ranging from 0.3 to 3.0 instead of 0.5 to 5.0.

TAKING THYROID HORMONE

This recommendation was meant to help diagnose and treat the 13 million Americans with a TSH of 3.0 to 5.0 whose fatigue and weight gain have been ignored. Fortunately, more doctors are learning to treat the patient instead of relying only on the blood test.

Still, in many cases, doctors are not aware of the new optimal range in TSH testing and still use the old scale to determine whether a person is normal. Even the major labs doing thyroid testing have not bothered to change the normal ranges for both diagnosis and treatment of thyroid disorders. The 13 million Americans whose TSH blood tests fall between 3.0 and 5.0 could represent the tip of the iceberg for this problem. Millions of people's lives can be dramatically improved by simply getting a trial of thyroid hormone.

In two studies published in the *British Medical Journal,* patients who were thought to have hypothyroidism (an underactive thyroid) because of their symptoms had their blood levels of thyroid hormone checked. The vast majority of these individuals had technically "normal" thyroid blood tests. In the next study, the patients with normal blood tests who had symptoms of an underactive thyroid (who might have been considered to have normal thyroids and not in need of treatment) were treated with thyroid hormone. Guess what? The large majority of patients, despite being considered to have "normal" thyroids, improved upon taking thyroid hormone (Synthroid), at an average dosage of 100 to 120 mcg a day.

Taking Thyroid Hormone Can Decrease the Risk of Miscarriage

In a study of 984 pregnant women published in the *Journal of Clinical Endocrinology and Metabolism,* those who got blood tests for thyroid inflammation (called an anti-TPO antibody) and took thyroid hormone if the test was positive (despite the TSH being "normal") decreased miscarriage rates by 75 percent. This could prevent more than 50,000 unnecessary miscarriages a year in the United States.

THYROID TREATMENT

Besides relieving the symptoms of hypothyroidism, treatment with thyroid hormone can have other profound effects on your health. The Hunt Study followed 25,000 people with different thyroid levels to see what their risk was for dying from a heart attack over time.

It showed that women with intermediate (1.5 to 2.4 mIU/L) or high (2.5 to 3.5) levels of TSH had a 41 percent and 69 percent increased risk of heart attack death respectively, compared with women who had TSH levels in the lower range of normal (0.5 to 1.4). Women whose thyroid levels were actually abnormally low (a high TSH over 3.5) had an even greater risk of heart attack.

Cardiovascular disease kills 2,800 Americans every day and many more worldwide. But much of this is preventable using thyroid and other natural therapies. In many cases, it's a better choice than taking toxic cholesterol-lowering medicines (called statins). These medicines only decrease heart attacks deaths (when used for prevention in those without known heart disease) by less than 2 percent.

In addition, statins can cause not only muscle pain but also the fatigue that drives sugar craving.

Prescription Treatments for Hypothyroidism

Most doctors prescribe T4 (Synthroid) to treat an underactive thyroid. T4, though, is fairly inactive until the body converts it into T3, or activated thyroid hormone. If the problem is only with the thyroid gland itself, prescribing Synthroid will work just fine. It may not be effective in treating other thyroid-related problems, though. Unfortunately, both clinical experience and research published in a 2004 study in the journal *Thyroid* suggest that most of those patients on Synthroid are unhappy with their treatment.

You may find that you do better by taking compounded thyroid hormone, which contains a mix of T4 and T3. Either way, you'll want to take your thyroid hormone on an empty stomach first thing in the morning or take half in the morning and half in the afternoon (or at bedtime). Don't take it within several hours of taking iron or calcium supplements, or you won't absorb the thyroid hormone. Your physician should adjust the dose to what feels best, while keeping your free-T4 blood test in the normal range.

Some people benefit from using pure T3 hormone (Cytomel). A standard dose is 5 to 25 mcg. Or you can try compounded sustained-release T3. After being on treatment with Cytomel for three to six months you may be able to lower your T3 dose or stop it entirely. If you feel better initially and then worse (beginning more than four weeks after starting a new dose), you probably need to lower the dose. If you lose too much weight, try to eat more and lower the dose (discuss this with your physician). This is a more complex treatment for complex cases, so find a holistic doctor who is familiar with this treatment and can guide you in when and how to use it.

Synthetic T4 (Synthroid) and pure T3 (Cytomel) are available at any pharmacy. A combination of the T4 and T3 hormones (or sustained-release T3), which works better for many patients, can be obtained from compounding pharmacies. One of the best is ITC Compounding Pharmacy (www.itcpharmacy.com). See appendix D.

All prescription thyroid treatments must be prescribed and monitored by a physician. Holistic physicians are more likely to be familiar with and open to trying these treatment approaches. Unfortunately, many doctors are trained to stop increasing the dosage of

Good News in Hypothyroidism Treatment

A ground breaking study published in the highly respected and reputable *European Journal of Endocrinology* (2010) showed that the combination of synthetic T3 (20 mcg) and T4 (levothyroxine) is superior to T4 only/levothyroxine treatment for hypothyroidism. 49 percent of the patients in this double-blind, randomized crossover study preferred the combination treatment, and only 15 percent preferred levothyroxine-only treatment.

thyroid hormone once an individual's thyroid tests are in the "normal" range, even if the dose is horribly inadequate for that person.

Do *not* let your doctor use the TSH test to monitor therapy once the TSH drops below 2.0—it is totally unreliable. Ask your doctor to only check the free-T4 level and to allow you to adjust your thyroid dose according to what feels best for you, as long as the free-T4 test stays in the normal range for safety. When using Cytomel or T3 at doses over 25 mcg a day, thyroid blood testing becomes meaningless and should not be used. Treatment should then be adjusted based on symptoms, pulse, and other clinical findings.

Natural Therapies for Hypothyroidism

For many people, natural thyroid glandular supplements are very helpful. Thyroid glandular supplies the raw materials needed to optimize thyroid function. The herb blue flag root, which is a thyroid balancer, can also be beneficial. For a combination product, check off treatment #24 in appendix A. Glandular supplements can be especially helpful if you haven't found a good holistic practitioner yet. You'll find qualified professionals in appendix C. Don't give up until you find someone you can work with!

It's also important to get the nutrients that are critical to thyroid function. Make sure you are getting iodine (at least 200 mcg a day), selenium (150 to 200 mcg a day, but not more than 300 to 400 mcg a day), and tyrosine (1,000+ mg a day). Iodine deserves special mention because it is essential for optimal thyroid function. My clinical experience has shown that many people whose fatigue is accompanied by a low body temperature improve when they take iodine. Take an iodine tablet containing 6.25 mg (2,250 mcg) a

The Value of Natural Thyroid

Over the years, Endocrinology Societies have published guidelines advising doctors to stay away from natural thyroid. Now, a new study in the *Journal of Endocrinology* (2013) shows that more patients actually prefer it: 34 patients (48.6%) preferred Desiccated (Natural Thyroid), 13 (18.6%) preferred Levothyroxine (T4), and 23 (32.9%) had no preference.

day for two to four months if you experience sugar cravings and fatigue, have a daytime body temperature below 98.3°F (36.8°C) , or have breast tenderness or cysts. Higher doses may suppress thyroid function (with long-term use), so higher doses are best used under a doctor's supervision. Check off treatment #25 in appendix A.

Understanding the Risks of Thyroid Treatment

If you have significant risk of angina, do an exercise treadmill test done before undergoing thyroid treatment. Risk factors include smoking, high blood pressure, cholesterol levels over 260, being over forty-five years old, or having a family history of heart attacks in individuals under the age of sixty-five.

If you have blockages in the arteries that feed the heart and are on the verge of a heart attack, in rare instances taking thyroid hormone can trigger a heart attack or angina, just as exercise could. Thyroid treatment can trigger heart palpitations as well. These are often benign, but if chest pain or increasing palpitations occur, stop the thyroid supplementation and call your doctor and/or go to the emergency room at once.

Perhaps you've heard that excess thyroid hormone can cause osteoporosis. There is no research we've seen that shows any increase in osteoporosis in premenopausal women, or even in postmenopausal women if they are on estrogen, if you keep the T4 thyroid blood level in the normal range. If you need to keep the T4 above the upper limit of normal, consider having a DEXA (osteoporosis) scan every six to twenty-four months. If this scan shows loss of bone density, lower the thyroid dose. If this is not possible, consider the highly effective osteoporosis treatment measures we discuss later.

Hypothyroidism is discussed in more detail in the books *From Fatigued to Fantastic!* and *The Fatigue and Fibromyalgia Solution.* You can also find valuable information at Mary Shoman's website, www.thyroid-info.com. Shoman is a thyroid expert, a leading advocate for thyroid patients, and the author of *The Thyroid Diet*.

Summary: An Action Plan for Treating Hypothyroidism

1. Use prescription natural thyroid hormone glandular to treat your hypothyroidism.

2. Alternatively, you can combine Synthroid with Cytomel or get a compounded mix of T4 and T3 hormone (in about a 4:1 ratio) as needed.

3. Optimize thyroid hormone with thyroid glandular and key nutrients, including iodine, selenium, and tyrosine.

4. Check off treatments #24, #25, and #25a in appendix A.

16

IRRITABLE BOWEL SYNDROME/SPASTIC COLON

Sugar addicts may have a spastic colon, also known as irritable bowel syndrome (IBS), resulting in symptoms like gas, bloating, and diarrhea and/or constipation. When type 1 sugar addicts run out of energy, it affects the hypothalamus and, in turn, bowel function. The hypothalamus is a control center in the brain for your autonomic nervous system. In addition to regulating sweating and blood pressure, it also causes contractions in your digestive tract. This long muscular "food tube" carries your food from your mouth through your digestive system and then out of the body. Contractions in your digestive tract are called peristalsis or bowel motility. When things are working correctly, these contractions convulse in a rhythmic fashion, starting from the top and moving along to the end of the intestine, where food is eventually expelled.

But when the hypothalamus malfunctions because of sugar overload, peristalsis becomes disordered. Instead of slow and steady rhythmic contractions, the large intestine/ colon often goes into random spasms, causing the symptoms of spastic colon. Some sugars, especially fructose, can directly trigger these spasms.

Normally, food that you eat should be digested and then come out in your stools within twelve to thirty-six hours. When bowel motility becomes dysfunctional, cramping can occur and normal amounts of gas can become painful. If the contractions are too fast and you get diarrhea, your bowels may not have optimal time to digest and absorb the nutrients from the food you eat. If the contractions are too slow and take longer than thirty-six hours to eliminate your food, constipation can result and your food may actually have time to become toxic.

These ongoing bowel contractions also push infections downstream into the large intestine, where they belong. If these contractions are faulty, infections can migrate upstream, where they can cause small intestinal bacterial overgrowth (SIBO). More on this later.

TREATING IBS/SPASTIC COLON

When treating IBS/spastic colon, the first step is to address yeast overgrowth. This process is covered in detail in chapter 8, which describes treatment for type 3 sugar addicts. Eliminating yeast overgrowth will often eliminate the problem of spastic colon in most people. But if it persists, you can take other actions to get well, including treating parasites and changing your eating habits by using Doris Rapp's Elimination Diet, which is also covered in chapter 8.

Treat Candida and Other Infections

In type 3 sugar addicts, IBS is due predominantly to bowel infections, especially yeast/candida overgrowth resulting from excessive sugar consumption. This is especially true in people who have associated nasal congestion or chronic sinusitis.

In any sugar addiction type, low thyroid hormone levels have a major effect on how well the bowel functions. If you have hypothyroidism, it's likely that you often have to deal with constipation, for example. An underactive thyroid is also a major contributor to SIBO and spastic colon. By treating candida and other bowel infections, as well as by eliminating sugars and treating the low thyroid, the problem will often go away.

The most effective way to eliminate spastic colon is to treat the underlying causes. Sometimes spastic colon is caused by a food sensitivity, such as to the lactose in milk or the fructose in sodas. More often, however, the culprit is an underlying fungal or other bowel infection. Once this is treated, the disorder resolves.

Unfortunately, no reliable test exists for fungal overgrowth, which is why doctors often miss it. How do you know whether you have a fungal/yeast overgrowth? As you learned in chapters 3 and 8, spastic colon itself suggests that treatment for yeast is warranted, and you especially need to suspect yeast overgrowth if you also have chronic sinusitis or nasal congestion. These also often go away when the fungal infection is treated, along with the spastic colon.

R℞ YOUR WELLNESS PRESCRIPTION - PART 1

☐ 1. Treat candida/yeast.

☐ 2. Avoid milk and fructose (i.e., sodas and fruit drinks) for ten days.

☐ 3. If symptoms persist, consider a seven- to ten-day elimination diet to rule out food allergies.

☐ 4. Treat symptoms of IBS with enteric-coated peppermint.

☐ 5. Treat for parasites if necessary.

☐ 6. Use special antibiotics when indicated.

Eliminate Lactose and Fructose from Your Diet

Besides kicking the sugar habit, it's especially important to stop drinking lactose (found in milk) and fructose (found in sodas and fruit drinks) for ten days. If you feel better, stay off the fructose (diet sodas are okay) and try lactose-free milk products. Even if you are lactose intolerant, you can still drink some milk. But because you don't have the enzymes to digest more than a certain amount, it causes gas. This isn't a health problem, but it is a nuisance.

Try an Elimination Diet

If symptoms persist despite eliminating sugars and lactose for ten days, consider trying Doris Rapp's food elimination diet in chapter 8 to identify food allergies. If symptoms persist unchanged after seven to ten days on the elimination diet, food allergies are less likely to be a cause of your problem. If your symptoms decrease, then add different food groups back into your diet slowly to see which foods trigger bowel problems.

Enteric-Coated Peppermint

To help with the symptoms of IBS, such as pain, bloating, gas, and diarrhea, it can help to take peppermint oil. But it's very important that you take enteric-coated peppermint tablets so the oil is released in the bowel where it can be beneficial, not the stomach. Research published in 2007 in *Digestive and Liver Disease*, the official medical journal of the Italian Society of Gastroenterology and the Italian Association for the Study of the Liver, showed that a four-week treatment with peppermint oil (two enteric-coated capsules twice a day) improved abdominal symptoms in 75 percent of patients with IBS.

Test for Parasites

If symptoms persist despite the steps above—especially if excessive gas or diarrhea is an issue—it is time to look for other infections. Begin with stool testing for parasites and bacterial infections, using a lab that specializes in stool testing, such as Genova Labs (www.genovadiagnostics.com), DiagnosTechs, the Parasitology Center, or Doctor's Data. Stool-parasite testing at most of the other major labs most physicians use is just too unreliable.

When dealing with parasite issues and treatments, it is best to be guided by a holistic physician or a naturopath in a state that allows them to prescribe what you need. For example, you may need a trial of antiparasitic medication if any parasites are found through stool testing. What treatment you need will depend on which parasite(s) are found.

TREATING SMALL INTESTINAL BACTERIAL OVERGROWTH

Bacteria belong in the lower colon, but when they move to the upper small bowel (small intestine), you get what's known as small intestinal bacterial overgrowth (SIBO). If you have chronic gas, bloating, cramps, and diarrhea and/or constipation that doesn't respond to the treatments above, consider getting tested for SIBO. SIBO may also contribute to food allergies and nutritional deficiencies.

To diagnose SIBO, ask your doctor to do a hydrogen breath test (HBT) to look for SIBO as well as lactose or fructose intolerance. (Each of these tests will need to be done on different days.) Excess bacteria make hydrogen when they come into contact with foods such as milk and fructose.

If you have SIBO, a special antibiotic called Rifaximin (550 mg three times a day for seven to ten days) can markedly improve spastic colon symptoms for months. This antibiotic is not absorbed into the body and stays in the gut, making it useful for bowel infections. Unfortunately, it is also expensive ($300 for seven to ten days). An older but cheaper nonabsorbable antibiotic called Neomycin may work just as well. It can be made by compounding pharmacies or purchased by prescription from Costco (less than $50 for a ten-day supply). Take 500 mg three times a day for seven to ten days. Combining Neomycin and Rifaximin may work best for constipation-dominant IBS. This has been shown in research done by Dr. Mark Pimentel, who showed that constipation-dominant IBS is caused by the bacteria *Methanobrevibacter smithii* which makes methane and puts your bowels to sleep. The combination of antibiotics works best.

The Relationship between Hypothyroidism and SIBO

It's also important to treat for an underactive thyroid (see "Hypothyroidism" in chapter 15), which is a main cause of SIBO. As we said before, slow bowel motility keeps your body from washing the bacteria downstream into the lower bowel, where they belong. Magnesium supplements, which pull water into the bowels and thus speeds the elimination process, can also be helpful in treating SIBO.

Use Natural Remedies to Improve Digestion

Instead of using antacids, try natural remedies to improve your digestion. You need a healthy amount of stomach acid because the acid kills off most infections that try to set up shop in the gut. When you don't have enough stomach acid, bacteria are more likely to run wild, which can aggravate IBS/spastic colon. Antacids reduce the amount of stomach acid, thereby worsening the problem.

R̷ **YOUR WELLNESS PRESCRIPTION - PART 1**

☐ 1. Take 550 mg of the antibiotic Rifaximin three times a day for forteen days or take 500 mg of Neomycin four times a day for ten days if the Rifaximin is too expensive. If severe constipation, take both together.

☐ 2. Optimize thyroid function.

☐ 3. Take 200 to 400 mg of magnesium daily.

☐ 4. Switch to natural remedies for indigestion.

Instead of popping antacids long term, consider using remedies such as the herb licorice and/or mastic gum for one to two months to heal your stomach. In addition, digestive enzymes will help you digest your food properly. You'll find more information about optimizing digestion in chapter 17.

Summary: An Action Plan for Treating IBS/Spastic Colon

1. Eliminate yeast/candida overgrowth, milk and fructose allergies, and parasites. For more information see chapter 8.

2. Use natural remedies such as eneteric coated peppermint to relieve the symptoms of IBS. Check off treatment #26 in appendix A.

3. If you are constipated, increase your fiber and water intake. If it persists after optimizing thyroid and treating candida, consider the combination of Rifaximin and Neomycin.

4. For bloating, take Mylicon tablets. Check off #27 in appendix A.

5. Treat SIBO with Rifaximin and magnesium.

6. Optimize thyroid function. (See chapter 15: Hypothyroidism.)

7. Use natural remedies such as Mastic Gum to ease indigestion. For more information, see the following chapter on indigestion.

ER

17

GESTION

addiction can wreak havoc on your digestive system, causing indigestion and acid reflux. 1 sugar addicts, for example, caffeine and the acids found in coffee (even decaffeinated aggravate both indigestion and reflux. The energy crisis that results from consuming drinks also causes the hypothalamus (which controls your autonomic nervous system) function. This disrupts the rhythmic contractions, or peristalsis, in your food pipe (which s from the esophagus to the anus) and interferes with proper digestion. When peristalsis es disordered, food stops moving in the proper direction. Therefore, acid and food can eflux back up from your stomach into the food pipe.

pe 2 sugar addicts are prone to indigestion because they are often stressed out, which leads eased stomach acid production. In type 3 sugar addicts, excess sugar consumption increases infections, particularly candida/yeast overgrowth, as we covered in chapters 3 and 8. Yeast n sugar, using it to multiply. The chronic use of acid blockers worsens your digestion further sing even more yeast to multiply and overgrow.

hen you factor in the other problems associated with the way our food is grown and ssed, you can see how indigestion and acid reflux can become a major problem for addicts.

THE BEST WAY TO DEAL WITH INDIGESTION

We need stomach acid to help digest our food so we can get the nutrients we need. But too much can cause acid stomach (gastritis or stomach ulcers) and aggravate acid reflux, which is when stomach acid moves back up into the esophagus (food pipe). Your esophagus is not made to resist stomach acid, and even a little bit will cause it to burn. When this happens, you reach for medications that turn off that stomach acid. The burning stops, and you think the problem was too much stomach acid.

Unfortunately, using antacid medications for an extended period can cause bigger problems. When you don't have enough stomach acid, your body is not able to optimally digest food and you can become nutritionally deficient. This makes it even harder for your stomach to make the mucous lining it needs to protect itself and can set you up for even more reflux. Additionally, in your body's attempt to make stomach acid (when you take antacid meds), it makes huge amounts of a hormone called gastrin, which stimulates stomach acid.

Consequently, as soon as you stop taking the antacids, your stomach makes massive amounts of acid, which causes terrible heartburn. So you reach for the antacids once more. In essence, you become addicted to the antacids. The information below will show you how to break your addiction to antacids and allow your body to produce the stomach acid it needs for proper digestion.

Why You Need Digestive Enzymes

Most of the enzymes we need to digest the food we eat are naturally present in the food itself. Enzymes are what a fruit or vegetable uses to ripen. These same enzymes are also needed by

R̷ YOUR WELLNESS PRESCRIPTION

☐ 1. Take two capsules of plant-based digestive enzymes with each meal.

☐ 2. Drink warm liquids (not cold drinks) with meals.

☐ 3. Take 380 mg of DGL licorice (not the sugar-free kind) for one to two months and then as needed. Chew two tablets twenty minutes before meals.

☐ 4. Take one or two 500 mg capsules of mastic gum twice a day for two months.

☐ 5. Take limonene to treat an H. pylori infection.

your body to digest the food you eat. Your body also makes enzymes to aid digestion of your food, but these were only meant to be *in addition to* the enzymes contained in the food; therefore, they are often not enough by themselves.

Over the past thirty or so years, most of the enzymes present in processed foods have been eliminated. That's because the enzymes in food cause them to ripen quicker. Food processors destroy the enzymes present in the food in order to increase the food's shelf life.

For example, an ear of corn may be good for a week or so before it starts turning brown and the supermarket has to throw it away. A box of cornflakes, on the other hand, has a shelf life of more than a year. Destroying the enzymes leaves the food looking good, but can also make it fairly indigestible. Not being able to digest your food then causes indigestion. Since food has become processed, we've seen a dramatic increase in indigestion.

Your digestive system uses three main tools to break down food:

1. Stomach acid

2. Digestive enzymes

3. Bile

Because the digestive enzymes have been wiped out by food processing, your body has to make more acid, and that acid has to sit in your stomach longer in order to digest the food. The acid can then start to burn your stomach (indigestion) and reflux back up into your food pipe.

Antacids turn off the uncomfortable symptoms, but they also turn off a key part of your digestive process. Without proper enzymes or stomach acid, you are left with only bile. Bile is what gives the stool its brown color and the appearance of food having been digested when you have a bowel movement. Unfortunately, your body's ability to glean nutrients from your food can suffer—and so can your stomach.

When you don't have the enzymes you need to digest the food you eat, you may experience gas, bloating, and diarrhea, as the bacteria in your colon digest the nutrients that should have been already digested and absorbed by your body before getting to the large intestine.

In addition, the poor digestion of protein can contribute to food allergies, arthritis, autoimmune problems, a weakened immune system, and even psychological disorders such as schizophrenia. These can occur as your body absorbs large chunks of proteins before breaking them down into their component amino acids. Your immune system then has to treat them as outside invaders and uses up energy digesting those foods that make it into your bloodstream. This can exhaust your immune system and contribute to food sensitivities. If you check, you may find that your temperature goes up about forty minutes after eating as your immune system struggles to make up for a weak digestive system.

Many studies, including a 1976 study by Drs. Singh and Kay published in the journal *Science*, have shown that people with schizophrenia improve when they are placed on a milk- and wheat-free diet. Milk and wheat both have proteins that, when incompletely digested, can trigger brain inflammation. As you can see, when it comes to symptoms caused by poor digestion, indigestion is just the tip of the iceberg.

Improving Digestion with Digestive Enzymes

You can improve your digestion—and your overall health—by taking plant-based (not animal-sourced) digestive enzymes. Plant-based digestive enzymes work in the acid environment of your stomach, where approximately 40 percent of digestion takes place. CompleteGest Digestive Enzymes are a good way to improve digestion, by both treating and resolving heartburn. Check off treatment #28 in appendix A.

While you are eating, drink sips of warm liquids instead of cold ones. Cold temperatures inhibit digestive enzyme function even further—your body's enzymes are made to work best at 98°F (36.7°C). Also avoid coffee, aspirin products, colas, and alcohol until your stomach heals and then use them in limited amounts.

Helping Your Stomach Heal

Taking DGL licorice can be powerfully effective in resolving your symptoms. Research shows that it is as effective as Tagamet—and it's healthy for you. Drinking two or three cups (475 to 700 ml) of licorice tea a day is another good option, and will also help improve adrenal function in type 2 sugar addicts. Don't drink licorice tea if you have high blood pressure, though. The DGL form will not raise blood pressure in people with hypertension and can be used instead. Gut Soothe (DGL Licorice) by Europharma helps to heal your stomach. Check off treatment #29 in appendix A.

Taking two 500 to 1000 mg capsules of mastic gum twice a day for two months is also highly effective. These remedies can be used separately or together. Because they help heal the stomach instead of just masking symptoms, they may take four to eight weeks to work in severe cases. Check off treatment #30 in appendix A.

You can use your antacids during that time if you want, switching over to Tagamet (cimetidine) as you feel better. Making this switch will decrease your stomach acid instead of totally turning it off. This allows your body to slowly ease back to its normal production of acid, and you can wean yourself off the Tagamet. After one to two months, you can stop taking the DGL licorice and mastic gum. If symptoms recur, begin this treatment again.

For many patients, stomach infections (*H. pylori*) can be a major cause of long-term indigestion. Your doctor can diagnose this with stool, blood, or other tests. Most doctors treat this with Prilosec combined with two or three antibiotics used simultaneously. A safer and often effective approach is to add limonene (such as Advanced Heartburn Rescue Therapy). Take it once your indigestion has settled down a bit as a result of using licorice and/or mastic gum. Limonene may initially aggravate reflux symptoms, but by killing the infection, it may give you long-term relief after a single course of ten capsules. Check off treatment #31 in appendix A.

Summary: An Action Plan for Treating Indigestion

1. Take digestive enzymes, plus DGL licorice and/or or mastic gum for indigestion.
2. Treat *H. Pylori* infections with limonene.
3. Try chewable antacids from Europharma.
4. Check off treatments #28, #29, #30, and #31 in appendix A.

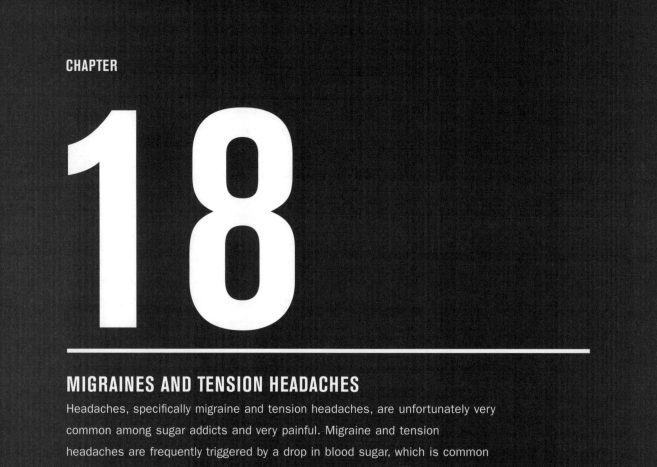

18

MIGRAINES AND TENSION HEADACHES

Headaches, specifically migraine and tension headaches, are unfortunately very common among sugar addicts and very painful. Migraine and tension headaches are frequently triggered by a drop in blood sugar, which is common in type 2 sugar addiction. When your blood sugar drops it can cause your muscles to go into spasm, contributing to both kinds of headaches.

Migraines: By the Numbers

Many people do not realize how devastating and widespread migraine pain is, but according to the Migraine Research Foundation.org:

- Nearly 1 in 4 U.S. households includes someone with migraine.

- Over 10 percent of the population—including children—suffers from migraine.

- About 18 percent of American women and 6 percent of men suffer from migraine.

- Migraine ranks in the top 20 of the world's most disabling medical illnesses.

- Every 10 seconds, someone in the United States goes to the emergency room with a headache or migraine.

- More than 90 percent of sufferers are unable to work or function normally during their migraine.

Food allergies to sugar and/or chocolate are also a common trigger for migraines. Because of this, many people find that their headaches decrease when they stop eating sugar and chocolate in particular. Why and how these foods trigger allergic migraines is unknown. Using the elimination diet discussed in chapter 8 is the best way to determine whether this is occurring.

Rapid fluctuations in estrogen levels, which affect serotonin production around your period or in perimenopause, are another common migraine trigger. If you get migraines mostly around the time of your period, or in the mornings before taking birth control pills, you need to prevent the fluctuating estrogen level. One way to do this is to use an estrogen patch for one week beginning a few days before your period is expected (e.g., a Climara 0.025 patch).

Although we know what may trigger migraines, the exact mechanism in the body that produces a migraine headache remains controversial. One theory is that migraines occur because of excessive contraction and expansion of the blood vessels in the brain. This is thought to be due to inadequate serotonin, the neurotransmitter that controls sleep and mood, which also plays a role in how blood vessels expand. Low serotonin also amplifies pain by increasing the pain neurotransmitter called substance P.

Migraine headaches usually last more than twenty-four hours if left untreated. Nausea as well as light and sound sensitivity can be present, too. Migraines are sometimes preceded by an "aura," which may consist of visual disturbances, such as flashing lights or blurred vision, but this doesn't happen to everyone.

The first step to stopping migraines is to kick your sugar addiction, which we discussed in part II. The second step is to use natural remedies that are highly effective at preventing migraines—and that can even knock out an acute migraine. In some cases, prescription medicines will be needed.

NATURAL REMEDIES FOR TREATING ACUTE MIGRAINES

Butterbur: This herb can eliminate and prevent migraines. Use only high-quality brands (e.g., Petadolex from Enzymatic Therapy or Integrative Therapeutics). Make sure that the product you use does indeed contain butterbur and does not contain impurities. Otherwise, it just won't work. Check off treatment #32 in appendix A.

Magnesium: Intravenous magnesium given in a hospital emergency room (if you get an open-minded doctor) or a holistic physician's office can effectively eliminate an acute migraine.

A study conducted in 1995 by noted headache specialist Alexander Mauskop, MD, author of *What Your Doctor May Not Tell You about Migraines,* involved thirty patients with moderate or severe migraine attacks. Half received 1 gram of intravenous magnesium sulfate over fifteen minutes and the other half were given a placebo. Those in the placebo group who were not better after a half hour were then treated with magnesium. Immediately after treatment, at thirty minutes, and again at two hours, 86 percent of those in the magnesium group were pain-free. Symptoms such as nausea, light sensitivity, and irritability were gone. None of the patients had a recurrence of pain within twenty-four hours. This shows magnesium to be far more effective than narcotics for relieving migraine pain.

NATURAL REMEDIES FOR PREVENTING MIGRAINES

Natural remedies can also be effective in preventing migraines. They may take as much as six to twelve weeks to start working, however, so the medications discussed below can be used while you're waiting for the natural preventives to take effect.

Magnesium: Magnesium is vital for an enormous number of functions in the body, including the relaxation of muscles and arteries. For this reason, taking magnesium in supplement form can also help prevent migraines. Research shows it's as effective as the medication Elavil. A study published in the medical journal *Magnesium Research* in 2008 showed that people who have migraine headaches who do not get a warning aura (e.g., flashing lights) had markedly fewer migraines when they took 600 mg a day of magnesium citrate for three months.

In a study published in the medical journal *Cephalgia* in 1996, patients were given either 600 mg of magnesium daily for twelve weeks or a placebo. There was a significant drop in migraine frequency in the magnesium group. A study published in the medical journal *Headache* in 1991 showed similar effects in women with menstrual-related migraines. Recommended daily dose: Take 150 to 200 mg of magnesium in the morning and again with dinner or at bedtime (use sustained-release magnesium if diarrhea is a problem).

Riboflavin (vitamin B2): Riboflavin also helps prevent migraines. A study published in the medical journal *Cephalgia* in 1994 followed migraine patients who were given 400 mg of riboflavin with breakfast every day for at least three months. By the end of the study, the patients had a 67 percent decrease in migraine attacks as well as a decrease in attack severity. This was later confirmed in a placebo-controlled study. Note that it can take six to twelve weeks for the riboflavin to start working. You may then be able to lower the dose to 100 mg a day.

Vitamin B12: Vitamin B12 can also decrease migraine frequency. In a study published in the medical journal *Cephalgia* in 2002, patients received 1,000 mcg a day as a nasal

Rx YOUR WELLNESS PRESCRIPTION - MIGRAINE PREVENTION

☐ 1. Take 150 to 200 mg of magnesium in the morning and again with dinner or at bedtime (take less if diarrhea is a problem).

☐ 2. Take 400 mg of riboflavin a day. After six weeks you may be able to lower the dose to 50 to 100 mg a day.

☐ 3. Take 500 mcg of vitamin B₁₂ a day.

☐ 4. Take 50 mg of butterbur (Petadolex) three times a day for one month and then 50 mg twice a day.

☐ 5. Take 2 to 4 Vetromega tablets (fish oil) a day for six weeks. Then you can decrease to the lowest dose that maintains benefits (or simply switch to eating at least three or four servings of salmon or tuna a week).

☐ 6. Treat food allergies with NAET (www.naet.com) or an elimination diet.

☐ 7. Take 200 mg of coenzyme Q10 a day.

spray. The subjects' migraine frequencies decreased by an average of 43 percent after three months. Recommended daily dose: 500+ mcg.

Magnesium, riboflavin, and B_{12} are present in high doses in vitamin powders (see appendix A, treatment #36), and this is all most people with migraines need long term. For the first six to twelve weeks, supplement with the higher doses indicated above (check off treatment #4 in appendix A and add Vitamin B2 at 300 mg). If needed, then add butterbur. For hard to manage migraines, you can also add in the other treatments below.

Butterbur: Butterbur is a shrub that grows in Europe, Asia, and Africa. A standardized extract called Petadolex was used in several placebo-controlled studies—including a study by Diener of more than 300 migraine sufferers, published in the *European Journal of Neurology,* and one by Lipton, published in the journal *Neurology*—and shown to decrease migraine attacks by 52 percent (using 50 mg twice a day) to 57 percent (using 75 mg twice a day) after three months. Recommended daily dose: 50 mg three times a day for one month and then 50 mg twice a day.

Fish Oil: Fish oil has also been found to decrease the frequency of migraines. In two placebo-controlled studies published in the *American Journal of Clinical Nutrition* in 1985 and 1986, patients with frequent severe migraines that did not respond to medication found fish oil to be effective. Recommended daily dose: Take 2 to 4 Vectomega tablets a day and give the treatment six weeks to see its effect. Then you can decrease to the lowest dose that maintains benefits. Check off treatment #34 in appendix A.

Glucosamine: In a study published in *Medical Hypotheses*, Drs. Russell and McCarty found glucosamine to be helpful in a small study of ten patients who took it over a period of four to six weeks. Recommended daily dose: 1,500 to 2,000 mg.

Coenzyme Q10: According to an open study published in the medical journal *Cephalgia* in 2002, coenzyme Q10 decreased the average number of migraine attacks per month from 4.8 to 2.8. Recommended daily dose: 200 mg a day. Check off treatment #35 in appendix A.

I save fish oil, glucosamine, and coenzyme Q10 for patients whose migraines don't go away with the other treatments in this chapter. For those of you who are tired of migraines, it's okay to do all of the treatments together and then start weaning from them after six to twelve weeks to see what you need to keep the migraines at bay.

Yoga for Migraines

A study in *Headache* (2007) showed the effectiveness of yoga therapy in managing migraines. Seventy-two patients with migraines without aura were randomly assigned to yoga therapy or a self-care group for three months. At the end of the study, headache frequency, severity, pain, and associated depression and anxiety were all significantly lower in the yoga group compared to the self-care group.

THE ROLE OF FOOD ALLERGIES IN MIGRAINES

Food allergies, as we said earlier, can impact migraine frequency and severity. Approximately 30 to 50 percent of migraine patients get marked improvement by avoiding certain foods. But most people with migraines are not aware of which foods are triggering their headaches. Food sensitivities are an even bigger problem in children with migraines. To determine whether foods are playing a role in causing your headaches, it is helpful to follow Doris Rapp's elimination diet as outlined in chapter 8. This strict elimination diet will make it easier to tell whether food allergies/sensitivities are present because your migraines will be triggered when you reintroduce certain foods into your diet.

Research published in the medical journal *Headache* in 1988 and 1989 showed that when people avoided the ten most common food triggers, they had a dramatic reduction in the number of headaches they experienced per month—85 percent became headache-free. The most common reactive foods were wheat in 78 percent of patients; oranges in 65 percent; eggs in 45 percent; tea and coffee in 40 percent each; chocolate and milk in 37 percent each; beef in 35 percent; and corn, cane sugar, and yeast in 33 percent each. Some studies also suggest that the artificial sweetener aspartame (NutraSweet) can trigger migraines and other headaches, although this is controversial.

You may find that instead of avoiding foods that trigger your migraines for the rest of your life, you can eliminate the sensitivities/allergies using a powerfully effective acupressure technique called NAET. (See page 111 and www.NAET.com.)

PRESCRIPTION AND OVER-THE-COUNTER MEDICATIONS FOR MIGRAINES

Medications in the Imitrex family still remain the first choice for many physicians when treating acute migraines. It's most effective if you do not yet have painful sensitivity around the eyes. If you use Imitrex in the first five to twenty minutes of your migraine before you get the tenderness/pain around the eyes, it will knock out the migraine 93 percent of the time. If the pain/tenderness around the eyes has already set in, Imitrex only eliminates migraine 13 percent of the time (although it still helps the throbbing). If you are one of the lucky ones who does not get pain around the eyes, then Imitrex can knock out your migraine at any time.

Imitrex can be a good choice, but aspirin, Tylenol, and caffeine in combination can be equally effective at knocking out a migraine for some people. You can find this in Excedrin Migraine or Excedrin Extra Strength. Take one or two tablets per dose, using a maximum of four to six tablets spread throughout the day if the caffeine doesn't make you too hyper. The dose recommendations on the bottle are fairly low.

Midrin, which is a prescription combination of three medications, can also be effective. Take two capsules at the onset of the headache followed by one capsule every hour until the headache is relieved (to a maximum of five capsules within a twelve-hour period).

Other prescription medications used preventively can reduce the number of headache days per month by an average of 50 percent. These include Neurontin, beta-blockers (Inderal—avoid this if you have asthma or fatigue), calcium channel blockers, Depakote, Topamax, Elavil, and doxepin. Using the natural remedies above, you likely will never need these medications for prevention.

Acupuncture Can Relieve Headaches

Acupuncture is another option to consider if you have chronic migraines and/or tension headaches. In two studies conducted in New York City and London, acupuncture was found to be a cost-effective treatment. In a randomized controlled study published in the *British Medical Journal Online* in 2004, 401 patients with chronic headaches (the majority having migraines) received up to twelve acupuncture treatments over a three-month period. A control group received standard care. Compared to those receiving standard treatments, the acupuncture patients had 22 fewer headache days per year, 15 percent fewer sick days, and 25 percent fewer visits to the doctor.

☐ 1. Take willow bark extract that supplies 40 to 80 mg of salicin three times a day.

☐ 2. Take 300 mg of boswellia three times day.

☐ 3. The sleep herbs discussed in chapter 6 can be very helpful for muscle pain as well.

☐ 4. Take two capsules of Midrin at the onset of the headache followed by one capsule every hour until the headache is relieved (to a maximum of five capsules within a twelve-hour period).

☐ 5. Take 50 to 100 mg of Ultram up to three times a day as needed.

☐ 6. Acetaminophen, caffeine, and aspirin (Excedrin Extra Strength) can also be helpful.

HELP FOR TENSION HEADACHES

Tension headaches account for about three-quarters of all headaches. They tend to both start and fade away gradually and are the result of muscle tightness.

When coming from the neck muscles, they cause moderate pain on both sides of, and across, the forehead. Occasionally, tension headaches from the muscles at the base of the skull are felt on the back and top of the head or behind the eyes.

To treat an acute headache, herbal remedies such as willow bark and boswellia can be very helpful, especially when combined with natural muscle relaxants such as valerian and Jamaican dogwood. In addition, there are, of course, the old standbys Excedrin Extra Strength, Tylenol, and Motrin. Other prescription medications that can be quite helpful include Midrin and Ultram. Chiropractic adjustments and bodywork can ease tension, too, and are useful in some cases.

Summary: An Action Plan for Treating Migraines and Tension Headaches

For Migraine Prevention

1. Use natural remedies such as butterbur (check off treatment #32 in appendix A) and magnesium (check off treatment #33). You may also benefit from taking fish oil (check off treatment #34) and coenzyme Q10 (check off treatment #35).

2. Take a good vitamin powder that contains riboflavin and B12. Check off treatment #36 in appendix A.

3. Try the Elimination Diet by Doris Rapp (see chapter 8) to see whether food allergies are contributing to your migraines.

For Acute Migraines

1. Take prescription medications in the Imitrex family as needed. Excedrin Migraine is as effective as Imitrex. The natural herbal remedy Petadolex (butterbur) can also eliminate an active migraine. One gram of magnesium given intravenously for ten to fifteen minutes will knock out most migraines as well.

2. Check off treatment #32 in appendix A.

For Tension Headaches

1. Use natural remedies such as willow bark, boswellia, and muscle-relaxing herbs in the combination supplement End Pain (by Enzymatic Therapy) or Pain Formula (by Integrative Therapeutics) herbal mix. Check off treatment #37 in appendix A.

2. Take the herbal medicine Curamin.

3. Use topical comfrey cream (Traumaplant) menthol (Tiger Balm) on your forehead and neck muscles.

4. Use prescription medications such as Midrin and Ultram as needed.

5. Over-the-counter medicines such as Excedrin Extra Strength can be helpful.

6. Acupuncture can be effective for chronic migraines and tension headaches.

OBESITY

You know that indulging your sweet tooth can cause you to pack on unwanted pounds, but you may not know exactly why. It's due to several factors. First of all, excess sugar, especially fructose (found in sodas and fruit drinks), can cause insulin resistance. This means that your body has to make more insulin to handle the sugar you eat. Unfortunately, insulin turns sugar and other calories directly into fat.

Second, excess sugar intake can both cause and be caused by metabolic problems that result in excess fat production. For example, in type 2 sugar addicts, excess stress initially results in elevated cortisol (adrenal stress hormone) production. High cortisol causes weight gain and also causes insulin resistance, which leads to even more weight gain. As the adrenals get exhausted and your level of cortisol becomes too low, the low blood sugar then drives sugar cravings. Eating more sugar both increases your calorie intake and produces insulin resistance. You eat a lot more in order to treat your low blood sugar, instead of simply eating because you're hungry.

A Daily Frappuccino Can Make You Gain More than 50 Pounds (23 Kg) a Year

For every extra 3,500 calories you eat, you gain 1 pound (455 g). What does 3,500 calories mean in real life?

- A Starbucks 24-ounce (680 ml) (Venti) Vanilla Frappuccino topped with whipped cream weighs in at 560 calories (with 21 teaspoons [84 g] of sugar). Drink one a day and you'll gain 1.12 pounds (510 g) of fat per week, or more than 58 pounds (26 kg) per year.

- A McDonald's McFlurry with M&M candies has 620 calories in each cup (12.3 ounces [344 g]). If you eat one of these a day, that equates to 4,340 extra calories a week. This translates to an extra 1.25 pounds (569 g) of weight gain per week, or an extra 65 pounds (29 kg) per year.

In type 1 sugar addicts, underactive thyroid function or hypothyroidism can often dramatically decrease the amount of calories you burn each day, causing you to gain weight. Conversely, when energy levels drop (in all types of sugar addicts), it can contribute to an underactive thyroid caused by hypothalamic dysfunction, which again will pack on the pounds. All this can occur even if your thyroid blood tests are normal. You can read more about hypothyroidism in chapter 15.

As you can see, sugar addicts go through many metabolic changes that will cause you to gain weight. In fact, in severe cases, when it turns into chronic fatigue syndrome or fibromyalgia, our research has shown people end up with an average weight gain of 32 pounds. The good news is that when you treat the underlying metabolic problems, and eliminate your sugar addiction, your weight can finally come down.

KEY ISSUES TO HELP SUGAR ADDICTS LOSE WEIGHT

If you find you still can't lose weight even when you avoid sugar and treat your individual addiction type, it's time to take a closer look. Here's what you can do to restore a healthy metabolism so you can finally lose the excess weight.

R̥x **YOUR WELLNESS PRESCRIPTION**

☐ 1. Get eight hours of sleep per night.

☐ 2. Support adrenal function.

☐ 3. Treat for low thyroid, even if your blood tests are "normal."

☐ 4. Take a good multivitamin.

☐ 5. Take 400 IU of Vitamin D. (See sidebar.)

☐ 6. If you have sinusitis or spastic colon, eliminate yeast overgrowth by eliminating sugar and taking 200 mg of the antifungal Diflucan once a day for six weeks.

☐ 7. Treat insulin resistance by eliminating sugar intake.

☐ 8. If your fasting blood insulin level is greater than 15 units/ml, ask your physician to consider a trial of 500 to 1,000 mg of Metformin a day.

☐ 9. Metformin will cause loss of vitamin B_{12} so be sure to take at least 500 mcg of vitamin B_{12} a day.

☐ 10. Take 1,000 mg of acetyl-L-carnitine a day.

☐ 11. Walk at least thirty to sixty minutes a day.

☐ 12. Get mind-body-spirit support.

Vitamin D Can Aid Weight Loss

In a study published in the *British Journal of Nutrition* (2008) that involved sixty overweight/obese women aged twenty to thirty-five years who adhered to a low calorie diet, those with higher vitamin D levels lost more weight and fat. The authors of this study concluded: "The results suggest that women with a better vitamin D status respond more positively to hypocaloric diets and lose more body fat."

Sleep Eight Hours a Night to Control Appetite

The expression "getting your beauty sleep" actually has a basis in fact. Not getting enough restful sleep can cause weight gain. Poor sleep causes decreases in the appetite-controlling hormones leptin and ghrelin, which means you get hungrier, especially for sugar. Inadequate sleep also decreases growth hormone. Growth hormone stimulates production of muscle (which burns fat) and improves insulin sensitivity (which decreases your body's tendency to make fat). As researchers at Laval University in Quebec City, Quebec, found, if you aren't getting enough sleep, you have a 30 percent risk of becoming obese and can expect an average weight gain of 5 pounds.

As you can see, getting the eight to nine hours of sleep a night that the human body is meant to have can help you stay young and trim. Think of it as the sleeping cure for weight loss. Herbal remedies can be beneficial if you have insomnia. (See chapter 6.)

Support Your Adrenal Glands to Cut Sugar Cravings

You can gain weight in two ways if you have type 2 sugar addiction: when you are in the stressed-out, high-cortisol phase and when you have sugar cravings during the low-cortisol, adrenal-exhaustion phase. If you are experiencing hypoglycemic episodes, consider taking an adrenal glandular that includes licorice.

You'll find information about combination products that support adrenal health in appendix A, treatment #5. See chapter 7 for more about treating adrenal problems.

Treat Hypothyroidism to Keep Weight Down

More than 26 million Americans suffer from hypothyroidism, yet less than one-third of them are being properly diagnosed or treated. This is the case despite most of these individuals having what their doctors mistakenly consider to be normal blood tests. *As long as your thyroid function is inadequate, it will be nearly impossible for you to keep your weight down.*

The symptoms of hypothyroidism include fatigue, weight gain, cold intolerance with low body temperature (below 98.6°F [37°C]), achiness, and poor mental function. Having even a few of these symptoms is enough to justify a therapeutic trial of natural thyroid hormone. If you do have hypothyroidism, taking thyroid hormone can dramatically improve how you feel and help you shed those excess pounds. (See chapter 15.)

Address Nutritional Deficiencies to Boost Metabolism

When you are deficient in vitamins or minerals, your body will crave more food than you need trying to get those nutrients, and your metabolism will be sluggish. This food craving can be caused by many different nutritional deficiencies, so it's most effective to provide overall nutritional support. A good way to get the nutrients you need is to take a good vitamin powder. You'll find information about a good brand in appendix A.

Stop Yeast Overgrowth to Facilitate Weight Loss

Fungal (also known as candida or yeast) overgrowth, as discussed in chapters 3 and 8, contributes significantly to both sugar cravings and weight gain. Although we do not know the mechanism for this, the excess weight often drops off once the overgrowth is treated and eliminated. The main causes of fungal overgrowth are excess sugar intake and antibiotic use.

Common problems caused by yeast overgrowth include chronic sinusitis and/or spastic colon (gas, bloating, and diarrhea and/or constipation). If you have either of these, you probably have fungal overgrowth. Treating it will help you lose weight—find out how in chapter 8.

Treat Insulin Resistance to Regulate Blood Sugar

Insulin is the hormone your body uses to regulate blood sugar. It's the key that opens the door so sugar can go from your blood into your cells, where it is burned for fuel. This results in increased energy. It also lets you burn more calories so that you have a higher metabolism and lose weight.

Unfortunately, many factors in modern life cause what is called insulin resistance. When you become insulin resistant, it takes a very high level of insulin to get the sugar out of your blood and into the furnaces in your cells. Excess sugar intake (especially of fructose found in sodas and fruit drinks) is a major cause of insulin resistance. High insulin levels caused by insulin resistance will force the body to turn carbohydrates into fat, and this is a major cause of reversible weight gain. Other contributors include inadequate exercise and hormonal imbalances, as discussed earlier.

A simple blood test, called a fasting insulin level, will detect insulin resistance. Although the normal range (i.e., you're not in the highest or lowest 2 percent of the population) is considered 5 to 25 units/ml, if your morning fasting insulin blood level is greater than 10 to 15, I consider this to be excess insulin production suggestive of insulin resistance.

In female sugar addicts with excess facial hair growth, insulin resistance may be coming from elevated levels of the male hormone testosterone. High or high-normal blood levels of the hormones testosterone and/or DHEA-S suggest this is occurring. This can cause weight gain and create a problem called polycystic ovarian syndrome (PCOS). This can then trigger fatigue and poor sleep, infertility (which is reversible), and a host of other problems in addition to weight gain. PCOS is severely aggravated by excessive sugar intake, but often responds well to treatment with Metformin and adrenal support, as discussed in chapter 7.

If insulin resistance persists despite eliminating sugar, increasing exercise, and optimizing thyroid, testosterone, and adrenal hormone levels, it is often reasonable to add in the medication Metformin. Recommended daily dose: 500 to 1,000 mg.

In women with PCOS who have an elevated testosterone level, it is reasonable to begin this medication and other treatments immediately. In addition to encouraging weight loss and decreasing sugar cravings, Metformin can reverse many of the symptoms of PCOS, including infertility.

Metformin will cause loss of vitamin B_{12}, so be sure to take at least 500 mcg of vitamin B_{12} a day (present in a good 50 mg B-complex vitamin and in the recommended vitamin powder in appendix A).

Take Acetyl-L-Carnitine to Lose Fat

Another major cause of weight gain is carnitine deficiency. When you don't have enough carnitine, it also forces your body to turn calories into fat and makes it almost impossible to lose fat. Simply taking carnitine does not adequately help, however, because it does not get into cells optimally. Instead, take 1,000 mg of acetyl-L-carnitine (which does get into the cells more effectively) daily for four months to boost energy and allow weight loss.

Exercise to Lose Weight

As we've said, eating 3,500 calories equals 1 pound (455 g) of body weight, so an extra 500 calories a day can cause you to put on 50 pounds (23 kg) a year. The good side of that equation is that burning an extra 500 calories a day can burn off 50 pounds (23 kg) a year.

Walking is a good way to begin (slow walking may be even better—see sidebar). Your weight times distance determines how many calories you burn walking. It is best to increase the distance before working on speed. A simple rule of thumb is that if you weigh 180 pounds (82 kg), you will burn around 100 calories per mile. Walking an hour a day can easily make you 25 pounds (11 kg) lighter each year until you hit your optimal weight. Then it will keep you trim while allowing you to enjoy your food.

Go Slow When Walking

Researchers at the University of Colorado at Boulder found that you'll burn more calories per mile walking at a very leisurely 2 miles (3.2 m) per hour than walking a moderate to brisk 3 to 4 miles (4.8 to 6.4 m) per hour over the same distance. In all, slow walkers experience a total energy expenditure of about 10 to 15 percent higher.

That's because when you walk slower, you're walking longer. You also don't have the momentum from already being in motion, which makes your muscles work harder. Walking slower also reduces the loads on the knee joints by 25 percent, which is important especially for those who are overweight, obese, or have joint problems.

Get Mind-Body-Spirit Support to Encourage Weight Loss

If you eat for emotional reasons instead of eating to meet your nutritional needs—in addition to addressing the reasons (above) that have prevented you from losing weight—you may need to look beyond your physical body for answers. That's because emotional eaters, compulsive overeaters, and food addicts eat (specifically sugar and white flour, in many cases) as a way to soothe unpleasant emotions such as anger, anxiety, depression, sadness, boredom, and restlessness. Using food in this way can lead to weight gain.

Fortunately, you'll find many self-help groups that are very effective at helping compulsive overeaters and food addicts. These include Overeaters Anonymous (www.oa.org) and Food Addicts in Recovery Anonymous (www.foodaddicts.org).

Summary: An Action Plan for Treating Obesity

1. Get eight to nine hours of sleep a night. If you have trouble sleeping, see chapter 6 for more information.

2. Support your adrenal glands with an adrenal glandular formula if you get irritable when hungry. (See chapters 2 and 7 and appendix A, treatment #5.)

3. Treat for hypothyroidism, if you have unexplained fatigue and weight gain.

4. Take a vitamin powder to alleviate nutritional deficiencies. (See appendix A, treatment #1.)

5. Eliminate yeast overgrowth, especially if you have spastic colon or sinusitis. See chapter 8 for more information.

6. If your morning fasting insulin is above 10, discuss with your holistic physician improving insulin function by taking Metformin.

7. Take acetyl-L-carnitine to address a carnitine deficiency.

8. Exercise regularly. Start a walking program.

9. Reach out for help and support from Overeaters Anonymous and Food Addicts Anonymous if you are an emotional eater.

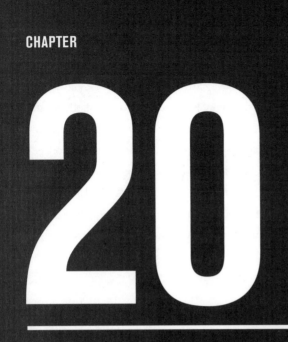

CHAPTER

20

OSTEOPOROSIS

Osteoporosis, or a loss of bone density, often occurs in sugar addicts and is a major cause of bone fractures, especially of the hip and spine. Why does this happen? First of all, the amount of sugar in 25 ounces (720 ml) of soda will increase the loss of calcium (a key part of what makes up your bone structure). Sugar addiction can also cause magnesium deficiency, which leads to a loss of bone density.

In addition, the initial increased cortisol production that occurs in type 2 sugar addicts also promotes a loss of bone density. Research done by Dr. John Yudkin, formerly a professor of nutrition and dietetics at London University, showed that a high sugar intake, especially of fructose (found in sodas), is associated with an elevated cortisol level.

For type 4 sugar addicts, low estrogen in women can dramatically contribute to loss of bone density. Although it's more common in women, osteoporosis also begins to occur in men as their testosterone levels drop. This is simply one more argument for optimizing testosterone levels in men and not ignoring andropause (the male equivalent of menopause).

Acid-blocker medications and antidepressants can also boost your risk. Sugar addiction increases the need for both of these medications. Finally, many sugar addicts are couch potatoes, and decreased exercise will cause loss of bone density.

TREATING OSTEOPOROSIS

The good news is that it is easy to treat osteoporosis safely, effectively, and naturally. The treatments below also don't produce unwanted side effects.

Take Calcium to Increase Bone Density

The best-known (but a relatively unimportant) player for increasing bone density is calcium. Take your calcium at meals and bedtime (e.g., 500 mg at dinner and bedtime) because it is better absorbed with food. Another plus: calcium taken at night can help you sleep better. Unfortunately, calcium tablets may increase heart attack risk. The best approach is to drink 1–2 glasses of milk a day and skip the tablets. If you do use tablets, they should have added vitamin D and magnesium, making them heart healthy.

Note: If you are taking thyroid hormone supplements, do not take the calcium within two to four hours of the thyroid hormone or you will not absorb the thyroid hormone. In addition, make sure that your free-T4 thyroid blood level is not above the upper limit of normal because too high a thyroid dose can also cause osteoporosis. (See chapter 15.)

Take Strontium to Build Better Bones

Strontium is amazing for building better bones. Don't worry, we're not talking about strontium-90, the very dangerous radioactive compound released during nuclear testing. The strontium we're recommending here is a mineral that's available in health food stores. Research shows that strontium is 170 percent more effective than the drug Fosamax for building strong bones.

A study published in the *Journal of Clinical Endocrinology and Metabolism* in 2002 showed that 353 osteoporosis patients showed a 15 percent increase in lumbar spine bone mineral density (BMD) over two years when they used 680 mg of strontium a day.

A placebo-controlled study of 1,649 osteoporotic women published in the *New England Journal of Medicine* in 2004 showed that use of strontium decreased new fractures by 49 percent in the first year of treatment. Bone mineral density in the lumbar spine increased by an average of 14.4 percent after three years. There was an 8.3 percent increase in hip BMD as well. Strontium can also reduce bone pain in osteoporosis patients.

Your body needs other nutrients, including calcium, magnesium, vitamin D, and boron for the strontium to work. Although these nutrients compete to be absorbed in your body, it's okay to take them in combination.

☐ 1. Take 500 to 1,500 mg of calcium daily. (In the form of a milk product or combined with magnesium)

☐ 2. Take 1,000 to 2,000 IU of vitamin D a day.

☐ 3. Take 500 to 600 mcg of vitamin K a day.

☐ 4. Take 200 to 400+ mg of magnesium a day.

☐ 5. Take 2 to 3 mg of boron a day.

☐ 6. Take 200 mcg of silica a day.

☐ 7. Take 340 to 680 mg of strontium a day.

8. All of the above can be found in combination products such as OsteoStrong plus strontium (in the Terry Naturally line by EuroPharma). Check off treatment #38 or 38a in appendix A. Take other nutrients critical for bone production: folic acid, copper, manganese, zinc, and vitamins B_6, B_{12} and C. You'll find these in the vitamin powder. Check off treatment #1 in appendix A.

☐ 9. Take 1 to 2 Vectomega fish oil tablets a day or eat three or four portions of tuna or salmon a week.

☐ 10. Supplement with bio-identical estrogen or testosterone to improve bone density.

☐ 11. If your problem is severe enough that you have osteoporosis, your physician may also prescribe a biphosphonate medication (such as Fosamax).

☐ 12. Walk at least 30 minutes a day or do another form of weight-bearing exercise.

☐ 13. Stop drinking alcohol or cut back.

Fish Oil Helps Decrease Osteoporosis

Fish oil from coldwater fish such as salmon, tuna, and mackerel can also decrease osteoporosis. Take it if you have dry eyes, dry mouth, or depression (all of these symptoms suggest fish oil deficiency). Eat salmon or tuna at least three or four times a week or supplement with a teaspoon of fish oil. I recommend you take 1 to 2 Vectomega pills a day, which replaces 8 to 16 fish oil tablets.

Hormonal Support for Healthy Bones

Make sure that your DHEA and testosterone levels are optimized because these hormones also can improve bone density considerably. In men, testosterone deficiency is a major cause of osteoporosis. Bio-identical hormones are discussed in chapters 4 and 9.

Even very low-dose transdermal (by patch) estrogen replacement therapy improves bone density in menopausal women. The findings come from a study of 400 sixty- to eighty-year-old postmenopausal women with thinning bones who received either the patch containing natural estradiol or a placebo. The results presented at the 52nd Annual Clinical Meeting of the American College of Obstetricians and Gynecologists in 2004 (held in Philadelphia) showed that women in the treatment group had improved bone density in their spines and hips and experienced less bone loss. The lead investigator stated that the ultra-low-dose estrogen patch offers a more natural approach to standard and unnecessarily risky menopausal hormone therapy (premarin) because it replaces circulating estrogen rather than increasing it in a toxic manner.

Take Prescription Medicines if Necessary

It's unfortunate (but not for you, because you're reading this book!) that except for calcium, most doctors only hear about expensive prescriptions such as Fosamax and calcitonin as aids for osteoporosis. Although these can be helpful, start by making sure you get the nutrients your body needs to build strong bones.

If you already have osteoporosis, you can take Fosamax or a related medication in addition to the treatments we suggest. The usual dose is 70 mg once a week on an empty stomach, taken with a full glass of water. It is best to take it immediately upon waking and then stay upright for thirty minutes so gravity helps it get past your stomach quickly (it can irritate the stomach). For those of you on the 35 mg a week prevention dose, you should be aware that the 35 and 70 mg tablets cost exactly the same amount—you can save half the cost by buying the 70 mg tablets and breaking them in half. (It is common for both low- and high-dose tablets of many medications to cost the same amount.)

Although Fosamax has been associated with jaw problems, the risk of this is lower than the risk of a bone fracture. Until your bone density improves from osteoporosis to the milder osteopenia, if your physician recommends it, combine the biphosphonate medication (like Fosamax) with the natural nutrients and bio-identical hormones mentioned here. The supplements and medications can be taken together to improve your bone health.

Exercise to Strengthen Your Bones

Although stretching exercises such as yoga and tai chi are helpful in general, when it comes to building bone density levels the most important form of exercise is weight bearing. This means means that your legs are supporting your body's weight. Weight-bearing exercises for osteoporosis include walking, climbing stairs, and even dancing. One theory is that weight-bearing exercise stimulates an electrical signal (called a Piezoelectric effect) that encourages bone growth.

Other exercises such as bicycling and swimming are great for conditioning. But they are not especially helpful for osteoporosis because you are not carrying your weight.

Walking as little as three to five miles a week can help build your bone health. Forty-five minutes to an hour of walking each day is even better. In addition, we recommend that people with osteoporosis avoid high-impact exercises such as jogging, which may increase the risk of bone fractures.

Walk outdoors whenever possible—that way, you'll increase your sun exposure, which enables your body to manufacture vitamin D. Vitamin D deficiency is becoming epidemic in the United States and is a major contributor to loss of bone density. It enables your body to absorb calcium from your food and move it into your bones.

Many nutrients also play a role in making stronger bones. For example, vitamin D and vitamin K have both been shown to increase bone density, as have the minerals boron and magnesium, which are critical for bone production. All of these are easily found in a good vitamin powder (see appendix A, treatment #1). In addition, excess alcohol may weaken bones and should be avoided.

Summary: An Action Plan for Treating Osteoporosis

1. Supplement with bone-healthy nutrients such as calcium, vitamin D, vitamin K, magnesium, boron, silica, and strontium. Take a good overall general multivitamin as well. Fish oil can also be helpful.

2. Supplement with bio-identical estrogen and testosterone to build better bones.

3. Take a prescription biphosphonate medication such as Fosamax, if essential.

4. Walk at least thirty to sixty minutes a day.

5. Avoid excess alcohol.

6. Check off treatment #1, #38, or 38a in appendix A.

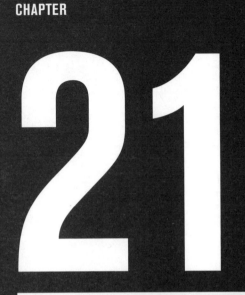

21

SINUSITIS

Chronic sinusitis is very common in sugar addicts, especially type 3 sugar addicts who have an underlying yeast/fungal infection (discussed in chapters 3 and 8). Eating sugar to excess causes the overgrowth of yeast. In turn, the yeast triggers an inflammatory reaction in the nose and sinuses. This causes swelling, blocking the drainage from these areas. Whenever drainage in the body is blocked (for example, when gallstones cause a gallbladder attack), a secondary bacterial infection will occur. Usually this is treated with antibiotics, but this just makes the yeast overgrowth worse and causes the sinusitis to become chronic.

TREATING SINUSITIS

Ingesting antibiotics turns short-term sinus infections into chronic ones because the antibiotics kill the good bacteria in your body, allowing more yeast to grow unchecked. This leads to more nasal congestion. A study published in the *Mayo Clinic Proceedings* in 2000 showed that more than 95 percent of people with chronic sinus infections actually had fungal or yeast growth in their sinuses, causing inflammation. For this reason, chronic sinusitis will keep coming back if you take antibiotics by mouth. However, infections can be effectively treated with antifungals and the correct nasal sprays.

Use Nasal Sprays to Attack Fungal Infections

Even chronic cases of sinusitis usually respond dramatically to yeast treatment with a special compounded nasal spray that contains Bactroban (a nonabsorbable antibiotic), the antifungal Diflucan, xylitol (which kills the bacterial and fungal infections), and low-dose cortisol to shrink the swelling. Bismuth in the spray will break up colonies of infection called biofilms, which antibiotics can't penetrate.

Use one or two sprays in each nostril twice a day, while you are also taking the prescription Diflucan to treat yeast overgrowth (see chapter 8 for more information). This is usually enough to knock out the sinusitis. You can, however, use this nasal spray long term and for recurrent infections, if necessary. The spray is available by prescription from ITC Compounding Pharmacy (www.itcpharmacy.com or [303] 349-5453). Simply have your physician ask for the "Sinusitis Nose Spray." Check off treatment #39 in appendix A.

Another helpful, over-the-counter treatment for sinusitis is a nasal spray containing colloidal silver. Silver is an effective agent against most infections. Liquid silver can even be taken orally for many types of difficult-to-treat chronic infections. Because silver is cheap in the very microscopic amounts being used, and it can't be patented, no one has considered it feasible to put it through the costly FDA approval process. This has made the remedy quite controversial. I recommend that you ignore the politics and try it. People have found it to be very helpful.

Squirt five to ten sprays of the Silver Nose Spray in each nostril three times a day for seven to ten days until the sinusitis resolves. For acute sinusitis, squirt 1–2 sprays in each nostril three times a day for chronic congestion. Silver also works well in combination with the prescription Sinusitis Nose Spray. Check off treatment #40 in appendix A.

Use Nasal Rinses to Clean Out Infection

If you have a sinus infection, nasal rinses can bring you relief. Dissolve 1/2 teaspoon (2.5 g) of salt in 1 cup (235 ml) of lukewarm water. Add a pinch of baking soda to make the solution gentler if it is irritating your nasal passages. You can even use plain lukewarm tap water without salt if you want to keep it simple.

Inhale (snort) some of the solution about 1 to 3 inches (2.5 to 7.5 cm) up into your nose, one nostril at a time. You can use a baby nose bulb or an eyedropper while lying down, or sniff the solution out of the palm of your hand while leaning over a sink. You can also use what is known as a neti pot to rinse your sinuses. You'll find premixed sinus rinses at health food stores or online, with directions for use. When you've finished inhaling the solution, gently blow your nose, being careful not to hurt your ears.

℞ YOUR WELLNESS PRESCRIPTION

☐ 1. Use one or two sprays of the Sinusitis Nose Spray in each nostril 2 to 3 times a day.

☐ 2. Use five to ten sprays of the colloidal Silver Nose Spray in each nostril three times a day for seven to ten days until the sinusitis resolves and then two sprays in each nostril twice a day until the bottle is used up.

☐ 3. Use nasal rinses to wash out the infection.

☐ 4. Take 200 mg of the prescription antifungal Diflucan daily for six to twelve weeks for any yeast infection.

☐ 5. Take a vitamin C powder to stimulate your immune system. Dissolve one packet under your tongue three times a day until the infection is gone.

☐ 6. See chapter 8 for more about treating yeast/fungal overgrowth.

Repeat the same process with the other nostril. Continue doing this, one nostril at a time, until your nose is clear. Rinse your nasal passages at least twice a day until the infection improves. Each time you rinse, it will wash away about 90 percent of the infection and make it much easier for your body to heal.

As a reminder, do not use standard over-the-counter decongestant nasal sprays like Afrin for more than two or three days because they can actually cause severe nasal congestion and chronic sinusitis when used long term. The approach described here will often clear up your chronic sinusitis within six to twelve weeks.

If you have a sore throat, gargling with saltwater, mixed as described above for the nasal rinse, will help.

Summary: An Action Plan for Treating Sinusitis

1. Use Sinusitis and Silver Nose Sprays to treat the yeast overgrowth in your nose that is fueling your sinusitis.

2. Use Diflucan to treat your yeast overgrowth (see chapter 8).

3. Use nasal rinses.

4. Take vitamin C.

5. If you have persistent chronic sinusitis despite treatment, read the book *Sinus Survival* by Robert S. Ivker. See www.sinussurvival.com for many helpful treatment tools.

6. Check treatments #39 and #40 in appendix A.

RECIPES FOR ALL 4 TYPES OF SUGAR ADDICTION

Good nutrition is an essential aspect of kicking sugar addiction and will help your body to recover and heal. Here you'll find a sampling of recipes for all 4 types of sugar addition and recipes for all types of sugar addicts. Start with one or two until it becomes a habit and then add more. Feel free to mix and match; many of the lunch meals can be used for dinner, and don't forget dessert! We think you'll be excited by these recipes that are good for you and taste good too! Enjoy!

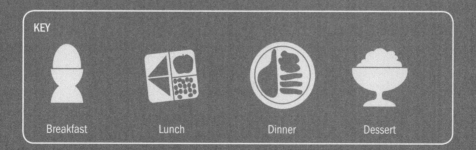

KEY

Breakfast   Lunch   Dinner   Dessert

RECIPES FOR
TYPE 1 SUGAR ADDICTION

These recipes are easy to prepare, which is a big plus in your on-the-go lifestyle. Over time, you will find that you actually prefer eating this way because it just tastes better! You're not looking to deny yourself pleasure. In fact, pleasure is good! You are simply learning healthier ways to enjoy your food. That makes this healthy form of eating easy to sustain, as it becomes a habit over the long-term. Remember, the best approach is to simply listen to your body by seeing what foods and combinations leave you feeling the best. Let's get cookin'!

GROUNDING GRAINS WITH BERRIES, NUTS, AND SEEDS

This is one of the most nutrient-dense, fiber-filled breakfasts you can eat to both balance blood sugar and give you energy throughout the day. This balanced meal of plant proteins, healthy fats, and low-GI carbohydrates also contains raw foods to help digestion. Flaxseeds are high in filling fiber and omega-3s, which help fight inflammation. Almonds are probably the best all-around nut for protein, with 6 grams of protein per ounce (28 g). They are also high in antioxidant vitamin E, energy-producing B vitamins, and calcium.

Other noteworthy ingredients include pumpkin seeds, a great source of immunity-strengthening zinc. Research published in the *Journal of Agriculture and Food Chemistry* in 2005 showed that they also are high in phytosterols, a plant compound shown to lower bad cholesterol levels. Sunflower seeds also contain high amounts of phytosterols and boost energy. The fresh fruits in this recipe are packed with healthy antioxidants, enzymes, and fiber.

1 tablespoon (9g) raw almonds

1 tablespoon (9g) raw sunflower seeds

1 tablespoon (18g) raw pumpkin seeds

2 tablespoons (24g) flaxseeds

½ to 1 cup (120 to 235ml) almond, rice, or cow's milk

½ to 1 cup (98 to 195g) cooked whole-grain brown rice (optional)

½ to 1 cup (115 to 230g) goat's milk or cow's milk yogurt

½ to 1 cup fresh fruit (such as [98 to 145g] berries, [85 to 170g] peaches, [81 to 161g] pears, or [75 to 150g] banana)

1 tablespoon (15ml) flaxseed oil

▶ *Soak the almonds, sunflower seeds, and pumpkin seeds in purified water overnight to enhance digestibility and increase enzymes. Drain first and place the soaked nut and seed mixture and flaxseeds in a coffee grinder or food processor and blend into a meal. Place in a bowl and add rice, if using, almond or rice milk, yogurt, fruit, and flaxseed oil. Serve immediately.*

Yield: *1 serving*

Each with: Calories 666.11; Calories From Fat 336.94; Total Fat 38.54g; Cholesterol 16.68mg; Sodium 149.26mg; Potassium 646.5mg; Total Carbohydrates 63.7g; Fiber 10.74g; Sugar 10.5g; Protein 22.62g

Health Facilitators	Nutrient Density Rating	Blood Sugar Balance Rating
Protein	High	
Fat	Medium	
Carbohydrate	High	Very High
Enzymes	Very High	
Antioxidants	High	
Fiber	Very High	

PROTEIN POWER SMOOTHIE

A smoothie for breakfast is quick and easy to prepare and to take with you on the run—something Type 1s love because of their busy lifestyles. This smoothie is nutrient-dense, with plenty of protein and healthy fats to give you long-lasting energy. Nutritional yeast is packed full of B vitamins and minerals, while the nuts and seeds add protein, good fats, and fiber, plus tons of vitamins and minerals. The milk and yogurt provide calcium to strengthen bones and magnesium to relax your nervous system. This means you'll have more energy throughout the day.

1 cup (235ml) cow's or goat's milk

½ cup (115g) plain yogurt

½ cup (120ml) coconut milk

½ cup fresh fruit (such as [73 to 145g] berries or [85 to 170g] peaches)

2 tablespoons (16g) or 1 large scoop of rice, egg, or whey protein powder

1 teaspoon to 1 tablespoon (2 to 6g) nutritional yeast (optional)

2 tablespoons (18g) raw almonds, (13g) walnuts, (16g) sesame seeds, (18g) pumpkin seeds, and/or (18g) sunflower seeds

2 tablespoons (24g) flaxseeds, freshly ground

▶ *Combine all the ingredients in a blender. Blend well and serve immediately.*

If you have milk allergies, avoid the whey protein powder and substitute coconut milk, almond milk, or water for the milk and yogurt.

Yield: *3 to 4 servings*

Each with: Calories 190.85; Calories From Fat 98.94; Total Fat 11.77g; Cholesterol 6.37mg; Sodium 66.96mg; Potassium 297.77mg; Total Carbohydrates 12.05g; Fiber 2.81g; Sugar 7.35g; Protein 12.9g

Health Facilitators	Nutrient Density Rating	Blood Sugar Balance Rating
Protein	High	
Fat	High	
Carbohydrate	Medium	Very High
Enzymes	High	
Antioxidants	High	

HIGH-ENERGY BANGKOK COCONUT CHICKEN STIR FRY

Coconut is an excellent source of plant-based protein and healthy fat, especially for vegetarians. It also gives this recipe a special kick! Coconut supports balanced blood sugar levels, and it provides thirst-quenching sodium, potassium, and calcium, which help keep blood sugar stable. Water also helps increase stamina and sustained energy. The almonds in this recipe may help you maintain a healthy weight, according to several studies. We suggest protein-rich quinoa here, but you can serve this rich and hearty dish with just about any whole grain, such as brown rice, buckwheat, or amaranth.

2 teaspoons extra-virgin olive oil or coconut oil

4 garlic cloves, minced

4 green onions, chopped

½ cup (130g) smooth almond butter

1 cup (235ml) light coconut milk

2 tablespoons (28ml) fresh lemon juice

2 tablespoons (28ml) tamari sauce (wheat-free)

1 tablespoon (15ml) fish sauce

½ cup (30g) fresh parsley, chopped

½ cup (120ml) purified water

1½ pounds (680g) boneless, skinless organic chicken breasts, cubed

2 heads of broccoli, including the stalk, chopped

¼ cup (30g) dried cranberries

¼ cup (23g) sliced almonds, toasted

1 cup (185g) quinoa, cooked (or any other grain, such as [195g] brown rice)

Yield: *6 servings*

Each with: Calories 398.17; Calories From Fat 175.95; Total Fat 20.35g; Cholesterol 22.67mg; Sodium 726.81mg; Potassium 586.16mg; Total Carbohydrates 39.87g; Fiber 4.95g; Sugar 1.97g; Protein 17.73g

▶ *Heat the oil in a saucepan over medium-high heat. Sauté the garlic and onions until softened and slightly brown. In a blender, combine the cooked garlic and onions with the almond butter, coconut milk, lemon juice, tamari, fish sauce, parsley, and water. Blend until smooth. In a large skillet, combine the blended sauce, chicken, and broccoli. Cover and cook until the chicken is cooked through, about 15 minutes. Before serving, add the cranberries and almonds. Serve with the quinoa (or another grain).*

Health Facilitators	Nutrient Density Rating	Blood Sugar Balance Rating
Protein	Very High	
Fat	High	
Carbohydrate	High	Very High
Enzymes	High	
Antioxidants	High	
Fiber	High	

TRYPTOPHAN-RICH TURKEY MEATLOAF MEDLEY

Turkey contains high amounts of tryptophan, a powerful amino acid that converts to serotonin, a "feel good" neurotransmitter that gives you a natural lift, making it less likely that you'll reach for an energy drink to do the job. You can also substitute beef and chicken, which contain tryptophan as well. Garlic adds delicious flavor and is antiviral, antimicrobial, and immune-protective. Served with steamed veggies or a spinach salad, this dish is wonderful eaten hot or cold.

1 tablespoon (15ml) extra-virgin olive oil or coconut oil (melted)

20 ounces (560g) lean ground turkey, beef, or chicken

2 large eggs

½ cup (40g) rolled oats

⅔ cup (110g) chopped onion

½ cup (123g) tomato sauce, divided

1 tablespoon (4g) fresh parsley, chopped

2 tablespoons (2g) fresh cilantro, chopped

1 clove of fresh garlic, chopped finely or minced

1 tablespoon (15ml) Bragg's liquid amino acid or tamari sauce (wheat-free)

Salt and pepper to taste

▶ Preheat the oven to 350°F (180°C, or gas mark 4). Lightly coat the bottom of a shallow baking pan with the olive oil or coconut oil. Combine the ground turkey, eggs, rolled oats, and onion in a medium bowl and mix thoroughly. Mix in 1/4 cup (62g) of the tomato sauce, parsley, cilantro, garlic, and Bragg's or tamari. Add salt and pepper to taste. Shape the mixture into an oval loaf and place in prepared baking dish. Pour the remaining 1/4 cup (62g) of tomato sauce over the meatloaf, cover with foil, and bake for 45 minutes, removing the foil for the last 10 minutes of baking. Remove the meatloaf from the pan immediately. Slice and serve with a green salad or steamed vegetables.

Yield: *6 to 8 servings*

Each with: Calories 218.61; Calories From Fat 101.05; Total Fat 11.25g; Cholesterol 142.46mg; Sodium 497.89mg; Potassium 436.22mg; Total Carbohydrates 5.8g; Fiber 1.34g; Sugar 1.36g; Protein 22.71g

Health Facilitators	Nutrient Density Rating	Blood Sugar Balance Rating
Protein	Very High	
Fat	Medium	
Carbohydrate	Medium	Very High
Enzymes	Low	
Antioxidants	High	
Fiber	Medium	

RESTORATIVE RISOTTO

This recipe is well-suited for Type 1s because it is so nutrient-dense. The rice provides protein and essential amino acids; the feta contains blood sugar–stabilizing fat, protein, and calcium; and other ingredients supply calcium, magnesium, B vitamins, tryptophan, potassium, and fiber.

3 tablespoons (45ml) extra-virgin olive oil (or oil from sun-dried tomatoes)

2 fresh garlic cloves, minced

1 small red or brown onion, diced

½ cup (55g) oil-packed sun-dried tomatoes, strained and slivered, reserve oil if desired

1½ cups (278g) brown rice, rinsed and drained

4 cups (950ml) vegetable stock or purified water, simmering hot

½ pound (225g) asparagus, trimmed and cut into ½-inch (1.3 cm) pieces

¼ cup (10g) shredded fresh basil, or 2 teaspoons dried basil

1 cup (150g) crumbled goat's milk feta cheese

1 tablespoon (15ml) lemon juice

2 teaspoons grated lemon zest

Freshly ground black pepper

4 cups (220g) fresh mixed lettuce greens or (120g) raw spinach

Yield: *4 servings*

Each with: Calories 592.16; Calories From Fat 222.94; Total Fat 25.4g; Cholesterol 40.58mg; Sodium 806.02mg; Potassium 725.2mg; Total Carbohydrates 79.98g; Fiber 8.17g; Sugar 6.46g; Protein 18.91g

▶ *In a large saucepan, heat the oil over medium-high heat. When the oil is hot, add the garlic and onion and sauté until softened, about 5 minutes. Add the tomatoes and rice. Stir gently, thoroughly coating the grains with oil. Add a cup (235ml) of stock into the rice and cook over medium heat, uncovered, stirring constantly until all the liquid is absorbed. Continue adding 1 cup of stock at a time, stirring constantly until the stock has been absorbed between each addition. Cook until the rice is tender, about 15 to 20 minutes.*

In a separate saucepan, bring 4 cups (950 ml) of water to boil. Boil the asparagus until just barely tender, about 3 to 6 minutes. Drain, rinse under cold water. Add the asparagus, basil, feta, lemon juice, lemon zest, and black pepper to the rice. Serve over a bed of mixed lettuce greens.

Health Facilitators	Nutrient Density Rating	Blood Sugar Balance Rating
Protein	High	
Fat	Medium	
Carbohydrate	Very High	Very High
Enzymes	Low	
Antioxidants	Medium	
Fiber	Very High	

SUPERCHARGED SPICY SALMON

Salmon is a super fish. High in protein and loaded with omega-3 essential fatty acids, salmon helps regulate blood sugar levels, quiets inflammation, improves circulation, and boosts brain health by feeding necessary neurotransmitters. Together with coconut, the combination works powerfully to keep blood sugar stable. The zucchini, carrots, and red onions in this dish are high in key vitamins C, A, B_6, B_1, and folate, as well as zinc, calcium, magnesium, and tryptophan, plus dietary fiber that all support metabolism, energy production, and overall health. Serve with a side salad, steamed veggies, or over a bed of steamed brown rice for extra fiber, protein, and nutrients.

1 tablespoon (15ml) extra-virgin olive oil or (15g) coconut oil

1 medium red onion, chopped

2 garlic cloves, chopped or pressed

1 can (14 ounces, or 425ml) light coconut milk, unsweetened

1 cup (235ml) chicken stock

½ to 1 tablespoon (8 to 15g) red curry paste, depending on desired spiciness

2 medium carrots, julienned

1 medium zucchini, julienned

4 salmon fillets (5 ounces, or 140g each)

Salt and pepper to taste

4 scallions, thinly sliced

▶ Preheat the broiler. Heat the oil in a medium saucepan over medium heat. Add the onions and garlic, sautéing until the onion is translucent. Mix in the coconut milk and stock. Add the curry paste and then bring to a boil. Reduce the heat and cook until the liquid becomes slightly creamy, about 20 minutes. Add the carrots and zucchini to the coconut milk mixture and cook until crisp-tender, about 5 minutes. Meanwhile, place the salmon on baking sheet greased with olive or coconut oil. Season with salt and pepper to taste and then broil until the fish turns opaque, about 10 minutes. Place the salmon on serving plates and spoon the sauce over the fish. Top with sliced scallions.

Yield: *4 Servings*

Each with: Calories 435.41; Calories From Fat 233.84; Total Fat 26.17g; Cholesterol 89.3mg; Sodium 426.05mg; Potassium 909.64mg; Total Carbohydrates 15.01g; Fiber 3.92g; Sugar 3.49g; Protein 34.36g

Health Facilitators	Nutrient Density Rating	Blood Sugar Balance Rating
Protein	Very High	
Fat	High	
Carbohydrate	High	Very High
Enzymes	Medium	
Antioxidants	High	
Fiber	Medium	

REFRESHING RHUBARB AND STRAWBERRY PUDDING

Try this delicious combination of antioxidant-rich fruits on a hot summer afternoon. Walnuts and almonds balance out the flavors and textures of the pudding while keeping blood sugar levels stable. Rhubarb and strawberries are both high in vitamin C, fiber, and calcium, and walnuts are loaded with omega 3 essential fatty acids—important nutrients to keep you off the sugar roller coaster. This delicious dessert tastes just as yummy at breakfast.

4 cups (680g) sliced strawberries

2 cups (244g) diced rhubarb

3 tablespoons (60g) maple syrup, or to taste

1 teaspoon grated lemon rind

2 tablespoons (10g) agar-agar flakes

1 tablespoon kudzu, diluted in 2 tablespoons (28 ml) cold water

1 cup (230g) yogurt

½ cup (50g) almonds, chopped

¼ cup (30g) walnuts, chopped

▶ *Combine the strawberries, rhubarb, maple syrup, and lemon rind in a saucepan and bring to a boil. Sprinkle in the agar-agar flakes and simmer until all the flakes are dissolved (about 7 to 10 minutes). Add the dissolved kudzu and stir until the mixture thickens. Transfer to a bowl or individual cups and refrigerate until set. Serve with yogurt and chopped nuts on top. Garnish with strawberry slices and a sprig of mint, if desired.*

Note: *Kudzu is a thickener and is available in well-stocked supermarkets. If you can't find it, substitute corn or rice starch.*

Yield: *4 servings*

Each with: Calories 290.23; Calories From Fat 129.47; Total Fat 15.44g; Cholesterol 3.68mg; Sodium 48.53mg; Potassium 743.9mg; Total Carbohydrates 33.23g; Fiber 6.72g; Sugar 22.4g; Protein 9.71g

Health Facilitators	Nutrient Density Rating	Blood Sugar Balance Rating
Protein	Low	
Fat	Low	
Carbohydrate	High	High
Enzymes	High	
Antioxidants	High	
Fiber	High	

RECIPES FOR
TYPE 2 SUGAR ADDICTION

The ingredients in these recipes have been specifically chosen to help nourish your adrenal glands and balance your blood sugar levels. For the best blood sugar control, try eating at least three meals a day, or five smaller meals per day, each with 20 to 30 grams or more of protein. Over the course of a day, you should also eat at least four cups of low-GI vegetables, one or two fruits, and several tablespoons of healthy fat. These recipes provide easy, delicious ways to meet those goals. Let's get cookin'!

GET-UP-AND-GO HUEVOS RANCHEROS

This perfectly balanced breakfast of protein, healthy fat, and carbohydrate supports your adrenals, which helps balance your blood sugar levels and keep your metabolism running smoothly. Corn tortillas are not only more nutritious than those made from refined white flour (they contain vitamin C, which supports adrenal gland function), they are tastier too. Fresh herbs, avocado, salsa, and cheddar cheese add flavor and stimulate your energy levels and your metabolism.

2 large eggs

1⅓ teaspoons extra-virgin olive oil

1 small tomato, chopped

1¼ cups (125g) scallions, chopped

¼ cup (38g) green pepper, chopped

¼ cup (65g) salsa or (36g) green chile peppers

½ teaspoon chili powder

¼ teaspoon cilantro, chopped

2 ounces (55g) shredded low-fat cheddar cheese

Two 6-inch (15cm) corn tortillas

1 ripe avocado, sliced

⅓ cup (77g) sour cream

4 sprigs of fresh cilantro

½ cup (130g) salsa

▶ Combine the eggs in a mixing bowl and beat with a fork. Heat the oil in a medium nonstick skillet over moderately high heat. Cook the eggs, undisturbed, for 2 to 3 minutes. Meanwhile, in a bowl, combine the tomato, scallions, green pepper, salsa or chiles, chili powder, and cilantro. Add the tomato mixture to the eggs and scramble with a fork. Reduce the heat if necessary and continue to cook until the eggs are set. Remove the pan from the heat, sprinkle shredded cheese on top of the eggs, cover, and let stand for 2 to 3 minutes or until the cheese is melted.

Place the tortillas on plates and divide the egg mixture between them. Top with avocado slices, sour cream, and cilantro sprigs. Serve with salsa on the side.

Yield: *2 servings*

Each with: Calories 747.65: Calories From Fat 379.18; Total Fat 43.58g; Cholesterol 451.76mg; Sodium 1340.01mg; Potassium 1903.58mg; Total Carbohydrates 60.37g; Fiber 16.71g; Sugar 12.8g; Protein 38.28g

Health Facilitators	Nutrient Density Rating	Blood Sugar Balance Rating
Protein	High	
Fat	High	
Carbohydrate	Medium	Very High
Enzymes	Medium	
Antioxidants	High	
Fiber	Medium	

FATIGUE-FIGHTING FLOURLESS CHICKEN FLAPJACKS

These nutrient-dense flourless chicken pancakes are not only delicious, they balance blood sugar too. Free from white flour, which is quickly converted to sugar in the body, this low-carb dish gets you off of the sugar roller coaster and leaves you satisfied.

1 cooked chicken breast

3 eggs

Dash of cayenne pepper (optional)

2 cups (110g) salad greens or (60g) spinach

½ of an avocado, sliced

2 tablespoons (28ml) fresh lemon or lime juice

▶ Blend the chicken, eggs, and cayenne pepper, if using, in a food processor until completely smooth. (The mixture will look just like thick pancake batter.) Spray a skillet with nonstick cooking spray and heat over medium-high heat. Pour ¼ cup (55g) of the chicken mixture into the skillet. You may need to spread the batter a bit so that it is not too thick. Cook for 1 to 2 minutes on each side (these pancakes cook much faster than regular flour pancakes, so watch them closely).

Serve over a bed of fresh salad greens or spinach and top with avocado slices. Sprinkle with lemon or lime juice.

Yield: *4 to 5 servings*

Each with: Calories 651.5; Calories From Fat 290.17; Total Fat 30.59g; Cholesterol 776.02mg; Sodium 424.93mg; Potassium 1292.59mg; Total Carbohydrates 13.54g; Fiber 7.37g; Sugar 2.63g; Protein 78.61g

Health Facilitators	Nutrient Density Rating	Blood Sugar Balance Rating
Protein	High	
Fat	High	
Carbohydrate	Medium	Very High
Enzymes	High	
Antioxidants	High	
Fiber	High	

MOOD-BOOSTING CURRIED QUINOA SALAD WITH TURKEY

This meal is high in both plant and animal protein, which stabilizes blood sugar and ignites neurotransmitters like tryptophan to lift your mood. Are you a vegetarian? No problem. Just take out the turkey and increase the quinoa. You can also substitute lentils or whole grain brown rice. The curry in this recipe adds exotic flavor, and the turmeric it contains is one of the most healthful of spices, improving brain function, speeding wound healing, and even fighting cancer.

½ cup (87g) quinoa

1 cup (235ml) purified water

¾ pound (340g) cooked turkey breast

¼ cup (25g) chopped scallions

1 tablespoon (15ml) extra-virgin olive oil

¼ cup (60ml) lemon juice

Fresh basil, chopped

Curry powder to taste

4 large romaine lettuce leaves

▶ Rinse the quinoa well and drain. Combine the quinoa and water in a 2-quart (1.9 L) saucepan, bring to a boil, and then simmer uncovered for 15 to 20 minutes or until all the water is absorbed. Fluff the quinoa with a fork and let cool slightly. Place the quinoa in a large bowl and add the turkey breast, scallions, olive oil, and lemon juice. Add the basil and curry powder to taste. Refrigerate for 1 to 2 hours to allow flavors to blend. When ready to serve, divide the mixture among the lettuce leaves.

Yield: *3 servings*

Each with: Calories 272; Calories From Fat 72.68; Total Fat 8.16g; Cholesterol 48.76mg; Sodium 1157.49mg; Potassium 583.97mg; Total Carbohydrates 25.76g; Fiber 3.13g; Sugar 4.82g; Protein 23.75g

Health Facilitators	Nutrient Density Rating	Blood Sugar Balance Rating
Protein	Very High	
Fat	Medium	
Carbohydrate	High	Very High
Enzymes	Low	
Antioxidants	High	
Fiber	Very High	

ENERGY-BOOSTING BLACK BEAN CHILI

If you're wondering how to replace red meat in your diet, try rich-tasting black beans. They are high in fiber and low on the glycemic index, which means they prevent blood sugar levels from rising too rapidly—making them an excellent choice for Type 2s and people with hypoglycemia or diabetes.

1 pound (455g) black beans, picked over and rinsed and soaked overnight

7 cups (1.6L) purified water

2 tablespoons (28ml) extra-virgin olive oil

1 medium red or brown onion, chopped

2 cloves of garlic, minced

1 small jalapeno pepper, diced

1 green bell pepper, chopped

2 teaspoons ground cumin

2 teaspoons dried oregano

1 teaspoon dried chili powder

½ teaspoon cayenne pepper

2 bay leaves

½ teaspoon red pepper flakes

28 ounces (785g) canned whole tomatoes, chopped (Reserve the liquid.)

2 tablespoons (2g) fresh cilantro, chopped

Freshly ground black pepper

1 tablespoon (15ml) fresh lime juice

2 cups (240g) grated Gouda or (200g) Parmesan cheese

1 cup (230 g) sour cream

▶ *In a heavy-bottomed soup pot, cover the drained beans with water and bring to a boil. Reduce the heat to medium and cook, uncovered, until beans are tender, about 45 minutes to 1 hour, skimming off any foam that may collect on the surface. In a large nonstick skillet, heat the oil over medium-high heat. Sauté the onion, garlic, jalapeno pepper, bell pepper, cumin, oregano and chili powder until the vegetables are softened and tender, about 10 minutes. Add the sautéed vegetables, cayenne pepper, bay leaves, red pepper flakes, tomatoes and their juices, cilantro, and black pepper to the cooked beans. Cook over low heat for 30 minutes. Add the lime juice. Taste and adjust seasonings. Remove the bay leaves and discard. Ladle the chili into bowls and top with grated cheese and a spoonful of sour cream.*

Yield: *8 servings*

Each with: Calories 264.06; Calories From Fat 38.44; Total Fat 4.4g; Cholesterol 0mg; Sodium 236.76mg; Potassium 1131.46mg; Total Carbohydrates 45.4g; Fiber 16.17g; Sugar 5.38g; Protein 13.57g

Health Facilitators	Nutrient Density Rating	Blood Sugar Balance Rating
Protein	High	
Fat	Medium	
Carbohydrate	High	Very High
Enzymes	Medium	
Antioxidants	High	
Fiber	Very High	

QUICK CHICKEN CURRY

This is comfort food that leaves you balanced and satisfied. It's perfect for those busy nights when you don't want to spend much time in the kitchen. To make the job even quicker, chop the vegetables ahead of time. Coconut milk is a tasty and healthy fat that helps stabilize blood sugar. Peas add fiber and flavor. Boost the protein by serving this over a whole grain such as quinoa or brown rice.

1 tablespoon (15ml) extra-virgin olive oil, divided

1 large red or brown onion, chopped

3 to 4 garlic cloves, minced

5 to 6 medium carrots, sliced into sticks

1½ pounds (680g) boneless, skinless organic chicken breast, cubed

1½ cups (355ml) chicken stock or broth

1 can (13.5 ounces, or 410ml) coconut milk

1 cup peas, (150g) fresh or (130g) frozen and thawed

2 to 4 teaspoons (4 to 8g) curry powder

1 to 2 teaspoons ground ginger

▶ Heat half of the oil in a large saucepan over medium heat. Sauté the onions and garlic about 5 to 10 minutes. Add the carrots and continue sautéing several more minutes. Heat the remaining oil in a medium saucepan over medium-high heat and sauté the chicken until cooked through. To the onion-carrot mixture, add the chicken broth, coconut milk, peas, and cooked chicken. Add the curry powder and ginger to taste. Continue to cook until the flavors meld and the sauce is heated through, about 10 minutes.

Note: You can add any vegetables you like to this versatile recipe. Broccoli and cauliflower are always good additions to curries.

Yield: *5 servings*

Each with: Calories 480.91; Calories From Fat 207.59; Total Fat 24.24g; Cholesterol 115.67mg; Sodium 427.92mg; Potassium 896.83mg; Total Carbohydrates 18.73g; Fiber 3.9g; Sugar 5.61g; Protein 47.52g

Health Facilitators	Nutrient Density Rating	Blood Sugar Balance Rating
Protein	High	
Fat	High	
Carbohydrate	High	Very High
Enzymes	Low	
Antioxidants	High	
Fiber	High	

HEALING HALIBUT WITH MEDITERRANEAN TOMATOES

The delicately sweet flavor of halibut pairs well will the herbed tomatoes and makes this dish a nutritional powerhouse. With plenty of protein and fiber; vitamins C, B_3 (niacin), B_6, and B_{12}; antioxidant selenium; magnesium; potassium; chromium; mood-boosting tryptophan; and omega-3s, this dinner will keep your blood sugar levels stable for hours and help restore your adrenal glands. Eat up!

1 tablespoon (15ml) extra-virgin olive oil

½ cup (120ml) chicken or vegetable broth, divided

2 medium red or brown onions, cut into medium slices

3 medium cloves of garlic, chopped

1 can (15 ounces, or 425g) diced tomatoes

2 tablespoons (28ml) fresh lemon juice

½ cup (20g) chopped fresh basil

2 teaspoons chopped fresh rosemary

2 teaspoons chopped fresh thyme

2 pounds (900g) halibut fillets, cut into 2-inch (5cm) pieces

Salt and cracked black pepper

Red pepper flakes

▶ Heat the oil and 1 tablespoon (15 ml) broth in a 10 to 12-inch (25 to 30cm) stainless steel pan or skillet over medium heat. Sauté the onion for about 5 minutes until translucent. Add the garlic and continue to sauté for another minute. Add the remaining broth, diced tomatoes, and lemon juice. Bring to a simmer over high heat and then reduce the heat to medium and simmer for about 5 minutes. Add the basil, rosemary, thyme, and halibut fillets; cover and simmer for about 5 minutes or until the fish is cooked through. Season with salt, black pepper, and red pepper flakes to taste.

Yield: *4 servings*

Each with: Calories 330.41; Calories From Fat 81.09; Total Fat 9.05g; Cholesterol 72.58mg; Sodium 372.4mg; Potassium 1285.19mg; Total Carbohydrates 10.82g; Fiber 2.31g; Sugar 2.84g; Protein 49.63g

Health Facilitators	Nutrient Density Rating	Blood Sugar Balance Rating
Protein	High	
Fat	Medium	
Carbohydrate	Medium	Very High
Enzymes	Medium	
Antioxidants	High	
Fiber	High	

CALMING COCONUT COOKIES

Can something that tastes this good be good for you? Yes! Not only do these cookies have great flavor, they are packed with fiber to stabilize blood sugar and full of vitamins and minerals like zinc and calming B vitamins that Type 2 sugar addicts need. Any nut or seed, and many fruits, will work in this recipe, so don't be afraid to experiment. For example, add 2 to 3 tablespoons (16 to 24 g) of grated zucchini to the wet ingredients to add moisture and flavor. If you can't tolerate any dairy, you can swap coconut oil for the butter without changing the flavor. The only sugar in this delicious treat comes from the fruit and the honey, which is all natural. Sweet!

1 egg, beaten

¼ cup (60ml) rice or coconut milk

½ cup (1 stick, or 112g) organic butter, softened

½ cup (120ml) coconut oil (melted)

½ cup (160g) honey

1 teaspoon vanilla extract

1½ cups (168g) coconut flour

1 teaspoon baking soda

1 teaspoon cinnamon

1 teaspoon sea salt

3 cups (240g) rolled oats

½ cup (60g) walnut pieces

¼ cup (36g) sunflower seeds

½ cup (75g) minced, peeled apple

▶ Preheat the oven to 375°F (190°C, or gas mark 5). Grease a cookie sheet. Mix together the egg, rice or coconut milk, butter, coconut oil, honey, and vanilla in a large bowl. In a small bowl, mix together the flour, baking soda, cinnamon, and sea salt. Slowly add the dry ingredients to the wet ingredients, stirring constantly, until you have a smooth batter. Add the oats, nuts, sunflower seeds, and apple, stirring gently until the mixture is uniform. Drop by spoonfuls onto a greased cookie sheet and bake for 9 to 12 minutes or until golden brown around the edges.

Yield: *25 to 30 cookies*

Each with: Calories 133.9; Calories from Fat 65.89; Total Fat 7.63; Cholesterol 0.03mg; Sodium 15.8mg; Potassium 49.71mg; Total Carbohydrates 15.16g; Fiber 4.58g; Sugar 4.93; Protein 2.23g

Health Facilitators	Nutrient Density Rating	Blood Sugar Balance Rating
Protein	Medium	
Fat	High	
Carbohydrate	High	Medium
Enzymes	Low	
Antioxidants	High	
Fiber	Very High	

RECIPES FOR
TYPE 3 SUGAR ADDICTION

Type 3 sugar addicts must be especially careful to shun sugar in its many forms—whether it is granulated sugar, high fructose corn syrup, honey, or white flour—to avoid feeding the yeast (candida) in the gut and encouraging an overgrowth, squeezing good bacteria out. To that end, the recipes in this chapter focus on low- or no-sugar meals.

Type 3 sugar addicts also must work to keep the immune system strong to defend against yeast and other infections that can require antibiotics, which also kill the good bacteria. In these recipes, you'll find important nutrients for immune health, including zinc; vitamins A, C and D; and selenium. The most important thing, though, is that these recipes are delicious, which will keep you and your family coming back for more!

MELLOW MILLET BREAKFAST CRUNCH WITH APPLE SAUCE

Millet is more like a seed than a grain and is easily digestible. Millet acts as a prebiotic to help feed the good bacteria that keep the intestines healthy and the immune system primed. Prebiotics are a special form of dietary fiber that nourishes the good bacteria in your gut. Probiotics are live bacteria, available in foods such as yogurt, sauerkraut, and supplements.

Millet is an excellent source of fiber and protein, which helps keep blood sugar levels stable for hours, and is high in B complex vitamins for fighting stress and helping you stay calm. Millet is also a good source of tryptophan, a precursor to the neurotransmitter serotonin that's important for restful sleep and even moods. A bowl of millet cereal with coconut and walnuts—which provide heart-healthy omega-3 essential fatty acids—is a wonderful way to start your day and ensure long-lasting energy.

1 tablespoon (15ml) coconut oil (melted) or extra-virgin olive oil

1 cup (200g) uncooked millet

3 cups (700ml) unsweetened, 100 percent apple juice

¼ teaspoon salt

¾ cup (60g) shredded coconut

1 tablespoon (15ml) vanilla extract

⅓ cup (40g) chopped walnuts

⅓ cup (33g) chopped almonds

½ teaspoon cinnamon

▶ *Preheat the oven to 350°F (180°C, or gas mark 4). Coat a 2-quart (1.9L) casserole dish with the oil. Combine the millet, juice, and salt in a saucepan and bring to a boil. Remove from the heat and stir in coconut. Return to the heat and add the remaining ingredients. Simmer for a few minutes, pour into prepared casserole dish, and bake for 45 to 60 minutes or until firm. Allow to cool before serving. Sprinkle with additional cinnamon, if desired.*

Yield: *6 servings*

Each with: Calories 340.97; Calories From Fat 123.42; Total Fat 14.68g; Cholesterol 0mg; Sodium 129.07mg; Potassium 335.89mg; Total Carbohydrates 46.38g; Fiber 5.33g; Sugar 17.74g; Protein 6.73g

Health Facilitators	Nutrient Density Rating	Blood Sugar Balance Rating
Protein	Medium	
Fat	Medium	
Carbohydrate	High	High
Enzymes	High	
Antioxidants	Medium	
Fiber	High	

HEALING HERBAL SCRAMBLER

Eggs contain choline, a nutrient important for neurotransmitter function that helps keep your mood lifted and your blood sugar levels stable and balanced for hours. If you can, choose organic, free-range eggs so you don't put the added burden of pesticides and growth hormones on your already-challenged immune system. The antibacterial, antimicrobial, and antifungal properties of fresh garlic, basil, and oregano will help keep yeast in check. This trio of herbs also provides potent antioxidant activity to strengthen your immune system.

4 eggs

2 large garlic cloves, chopped

1 teaspoon chopped fresh oregano

½ teaspoon chopped fresh basil

Pinch of cayenne pepper

Salt

2 to 3 finely chopped scallions

1 tablespoon (15ml) extra-virgin olive oil

2 cups (110g) mixed lettuce greens, (94g) romaine lettuce, or (60g) spinach

▶ Whisk the eggs in a medium bowl with the garlic, oregano, basil, cayenne pepper, and salt. Stir in the scallions. Heat the olive oil in medium skillet over medium heat. Pour in the egg mixture and scramble with a spatula, cooking until eggs reach the desired doneness. Serve over mixed lettuce greens, romaine lettuce, or spinach.

Yield: *2 servings*

Each with: Calories 220.14; Calories From Fat 150.76; Total Fat 16.87g; Cholesterol 423mg; Sodium 166.91mg; Potassium 362.76mg; Total Carbohydrates 4.17g; Fiber 1.34g; Sugar 1.3g; Protein 13.95g

Health Facilitators	Nutrient Density Rating	Blood Sugar Balance Rating
Protein	High	
Fat	Medium	
Carbohydrate	Medium	Very High
Enzymes	Medium	
Antioxidants	Medium	
Fiber	Medium	

BLOOD SUGAR–BALANCING BUCKWHEAT WITH CABBAGE AND CORN

Energizing and nutritious, buckwheat is a cereal grain that is rich in flavonoids, which protect against disease by extending the action of vitamin C. Vitamin C, a powerful antioxidant, improves adrenal gland function, which boosts cortisol production and in turn improves your body's stress-coping abilities. Buckwheat also contains protein and fiber, which help keep blood sugar levels stable. Cabbage is rich in fiber and sulfur, making it a potent ally when it comes to fighting against bacterial infections such as yeast and fungus. It is also abundant in vitamin C and, combined with zesty horseradish, onions, and herbs, will boost your immune system and rev up your metabolism.

2 tablespoons (28ml) extra-virgin olive oil, (28g) coconut oil, or (28ml) ghee

3 cups (270g) chopped cabbage (preferably savoy)

2 cups (308g) corn kernels

1 large red or brown onion, chopped

½ of a red bell pepper, minced

4 cups (950ml) vegetable stock or purified water

1 teaspoon sea salt

¼ teaspoon freshly ground black pepper

1 teaspoon mixed herbs, such as oregano, dill, and basil

2 cups (330g) roasted buckwheat groats

½ cup (30g) chopped parsley

1 teaspoon horseradish (optional)

▶ Heat the oil in a 2-quart (1.9 L) saucepan over medium-high heat; when hot, sauté the cabbage, corn, onion, and red bell pepper. Add the stock or water, salt, pepper, and mixed herbs and bring to a rolling boil. Add the buckwheat and simmer for 20 minutes. Turn off the heat and fold in the parsley and horseradish. Let it sit, covered, for 10 minutes. Serve hot.

Yield: *6 servings*

Each with: Calories 353.91; Calories From Fat 74.32; Total Fat 8.41g; Cholesterol 4.8mg; Sodium 699.07mg; Potassium 642.48mg; Total Carbohydrates 62.18g; Fiber 8.87g; Sugar 6.48g; Protein 13.08g

Health Facilitators	Nutrient Density Rating	Blood Sugar Balance Rating
Protein	High	
Fat	Medium	
Carbohydrate	High	Very High
Enzymes	Low	
Antioxidants	High	
Fiber	High	

SUSTAINING SHRIMP CREOLE

A delicious and wonderful combination of tangy taste and crunchy texture, this nutritious dish is bound to delight with every bite. High-protein shrimp balance blood sugar and contain tryptophan, omega-3s, selenium, vitamin D, B$_{12}$, iron, zinc, and magnesium, which lift mood and help you stay calm in the face of stress. Peppers are excellent sources of vitamin C and vitamin A, two powerful antioxidants that work to neutralize free radicals and give your body a boost in energy. Peppers are also an excellent source of vitamins D and B$_{12}$, which benefit your immune system. Toss into the mix the lycopene-laden tomatoes, which help protect against breast, prostate, and intestinal cancers, especially when consumed with healthy fats such as avocado and coconut or olive oil, and you have one tantalizing and healthful dish.

4 teaspoons (20 ml) extra-virgin olive oil or (20g) coconut oil

½ cup (75g) chopped green bell pepper

½ cup (50g) chopped celery

½ cup (80g) chopped red or brown onion

1 garlic clove, minced

1 can (28 ounces, or 805g) whole tomatoes, chopped and undrained

¼ teaspoon red pepper flakes

6 black olives, chopped

1 bay leaf

½ teaspoon finely chopped thyme

20 medium shrimp, peeled and deveined

2 cups (390g) cooked brown rice

½ cup peas, (75g) fresh or (65g) frozen and thawed

½ of an avocado, chopped

▶ *In a medium saucepan, heat the oil over medium heat. Add the green bell pepper, celery, onion, and garlic and cook about 5 minutes or until tender. Add the tomatoes and their liquid, red pepper flakes, olives, bay leaf, and thyme; bring to a boil. Reduce the heat to low and simmer, uncovered, about 30 minutes or until reduced slightly, stirring often. Add the shrimp and cook until the shrimp turns pink, about 4 minutes longer. Remove the bay leaf and discard. Serve over cooked brown rice with peas and chopped avocado.*

Yield: *4 servings*

Each with: Calories 311.98; Calories From Fat 91.55; Total Fat 10.63g; Cholesterol 45.6mg; Sodium 635.62mg; Potassium 759.79mg; Total Carbohydrates 44.89g; Fiber 7.65g; Sugar 10.97g; Protein 12.58g

Health Facilitators	Nutrient Density Rating	Blood Sugar Balance Rating
Protein	High	
Fat	Medium	
Carbohydrate	High	Very High
Enzymes	Medium	
Antioxidants	High	
Fiber	High	

ZESTY ZUCCHINI AND CHICKEN BAKE

Zucchini are an excellent source of vitamins C and A, both of which provide excellent protection from yeast overgrowth. Zucchini also contain immune boosters such as the minerals potassium, copper, and magnesium. This dish offers healthy amounts of lean protein from chicken and nutritious herbs that are pleasing to the palate. Pine nuts add crunch and extra protein, and fiber-rich brown rice keeps you satisfied for hours.

2 teaspoons extra-virgin olive oil or coconut oil

2 garlic cloves, minced

1 pound (455g) boneless, skinless chicken breasts

15 ounces (425g) organic tomato sauce

2 cups (240g) julienned zucchini

1 tablespoon (3g) chopped basil

1 tablespoon (4g) chopped oregano

1 tablespoon (2g) chopped thyme

1 tablespoon (6g) grated lemon peel

1 cup (195g) cooked brown rice

4 teaspoons (12g) pine nuts

▶ Preheat the oven to 375°F (190°C, or gas mark 5). Heat the oil in a large skillet over medium-high heat and sauté garlic for 30 seconds. Add the chicken, cover, reduce the heat, and cook for 30 minutes. Spray a 9 x 13-inch (23 x 33cm) baking dish with nonstick cooking spray. Pour the tomato sauce into the prepared dish. Place the zucchini, basil, oregano, thyme, and chicken on top of the tomato sauce. Sprinkle the lemon peel over the top. Cover with foil and bake for 30 minutes. Serve over brown rice and top with pine nuts.

Yield: *4 servings*

Each with: Calories 268.56; Calories From Fat 59.83; Total Fat 6.16g; Cholesterol 68mg; Sodium 643.83mg; Potassium 733.61mg; Total Carbohydrates 21.71g; Fiber 4.59g; Sugar 6.18g; Protein 31.23g

Health Facilitators	Nutrient Density Rating	Blood Sugar Balance Rating
Protein	High	
Fat	Medium	
Carbohydrate	Medium	Very High
Enzymes	Low	
Antioxidants	High	
Fiber	High	

CHERRY YOGURT FREEZE

Cherries are considered a "super"' fruit by many health experts because of the amount of disease-fighting antioxidants, vitamins, and minerals they contain. Cherries are the perfect fruit for Type 3 sugar addicts because they are low in sugar, and their high fiber content keeps blood sugar stable. Combine cherries' potassium, magnesium, folate, and vitamin C with yeast-fighting yogurt, and this dessert is a smart and delicious choice.

2 cups (310g) cherries, fresh or frozen and thawed

1 cup (230g) plain low-fat yogurt

2 teaspoons vanilla extract, or more to taste

Freshly grated nutmeg

2 to 3 tablespoons (16 to 24g) chopped walnuts

▶ *Freeze the cherries for several hours or overnight. Place the yogurt and vanilla in a food processor or blender and add the cherries. Process until almost smooth. Then process for several seconds until the mixture is completely smooth. Add nutmeg to taste, add more vanilla, if desired, and serve garnished with chopped walnuts. You may also hold in the freezer for up to 2 hours (it will become too hard if frozen any longer).*

Yield: *2 servings*

Each with: Calories 225.25; Calories From Fat 59.85; Total Fat 7.07g; Cholesterol 7.35mg; Sodium 86.28mg; Potassium 632.29mg; Total Carbohydrates 32.28g; Fiber 3.4g; Sugar 27.04g; Protein 9.04g

Health Facilitators	Nutrient Density Rating	Blood Sugar Balance Rating
Protein	Low	
Fat	Low	
Carbohydrate	High	Very High
Enzymes	Very High	
Antioxidants	Very High	
Fiber	Very High	

RECIPES FOR
TYPE 4 SUGAR ADDICTION

When hormones are out of balance during PMS, perimenopause, menopause, and andropause (male menopause), it can cause sugar cravings to soar. In order to stop Type 4 sugar addiction, we start with a healthy diet. These recipes have been created specifically to address the issues related to Type 4 sugar personality—they will keep your blood sugar levels stable, your hormones balanced, and you, healthy. Use them in combination with the bio-identical hormones and natural remedies described in chapter 10 to heal your body and feel better than ever before!

MIGHTY MEDITERRANEAN FRITTATA

The health benefits of broccoli and spinach make them mealtime winners, especially when it comes to keeping hormones balanced. Both are loaded with antioxidants, vitamin C, folic acid, and magnesium to nourish and support healthy hormone levels. Plus, the high-fiber variety of vegetables helps stabilize blood sugar levels.

1 tablespoon (15ml) olive oil, (14g) butter, or (15ml) ghee

2 broccoli crowns, cut into bite-sized pieces

1 medium yellow bell pepper, chopped

1 medium red bell pepper, chopped

2 cups (60g) chopped spinach

½ cup (50g) pitted and halved ripe olives

6 eggs, lightly beaten

½ cup (120ml) rice, almond, goat, or cow's milk

2 tablespoons (6g) chopped fresh basil or 1 teaspoon dried basil

1 teaspoon dried oregano

Sea salt and pepper

1 to 2 tablespoons (5 to 10g) finely grated Parmesan cheese

¼ cup (35g) finely ground cashews

▶ Preheat the oven to 350°F (180°C, or gas mark 4). Grease a 9-inch (23 cm) round pan with the butter or oil. Evenly arrange the broccoli, yellow and red bell peppers, spinach, and olives in the pan. Beat together the eggs, milk, basil, oregano, and salt and pepper to taste in a small bowl and pour over the vegetables. Bake for 35 to 40 minutes or until the center has set. Broil for the last two minutes to brown the top. Cool, slice into wedges, and serve warm or cold garnished with Parmesan cheese and ground cashews.

Yield: *4 servings*

Each with: Calories 334.77; Calories From Fat 223.62; Total Fat 25.71g; Cholesterol 320.79mg; Sodium 396.88mg; Potassium 396.52mg; Total Carbohydrates 13.82g; Fiber 3.88g; Sugar 4.11g; Protein 15.15g

Health Facilitators	Nutrient Density Rating	Blood Sugar Balance Rating
Protein	High	
Fat	Medium	
Carbohydrate	High	Very High
Enzymes	Low	
Antioxidants	High	
Fiber	High	

ENERGY-GIVING GRANOLA

This simple-to-make version of an old favorite will satisfy your sweet tooth and keep your blood sugar levels stable at the same time. The addition of omega-3-rich walnuts and flaxseed oil feed your brain cells as well as balance your hormones, and coconut oil boasts additional healing essential fatty acids. Sunflower seeds are loaded with zinc, which boosts your immune system, while the raw oats are full of filling fiber to keep your digestive system working properly.

6 cups (480g) rolled oats

1¼ cups (120g) unsweetened chopped coconut

½ cup (50g) chopped almonds

½ cup (60g) chopped walnuts

1 cup (145g) raw, shelled sunflower seeds

½ cup (72g) sesame seeds

Dash of cinnamon

Pinch of salt

½ cup (160g) raw honey

½ cup (115g) organic coconut oil

2 to 3 tablespoons (28 to 45ml) flaxseed oil

▶ *Preheat the oven to 325°F (170°C, or gas mark 3). Mix the oats, coconut, almonds, walnuts, sunflower seeds, sesame seeds, cinnamon and salt together in a large bowl. Combine the honey and coconut oil in a saucepan over medium heat and heat to a thin liquid. Pour over the dry ingredients and mix well. Spread onto a baking pan and flatten with moist hands. Bake for 15 to 20 minutes. Cool and store in an airtight container. Drizzle with flaxseed oil and serve with almond or rice milk and/or fresh fruit.*

Yield: *6 to 8 servings*

Each with: Calories 981.88; Calories From Fat 602.9; Total Fat 71.01g; Cholesterol 0mg; Sodium 60.74mg; Potassium 607.37mg; Total Carbohydrates 76.74g; Fiber 16.9g; Sugar 21.86g; Protein 20.18g;

Health Facilitators	Nutrient Density Rating	Blood Sugar Balance Rating
Protein	Medium	
Fat	High	
Carbohydrate	High	Very High
Enzymes	High	
Antioxidants	High	
Fiber	Very High	

SATISFYING TEX-MEX SALAD

A truly unique blend of Southwest cuisine and south-of-the-border ingredients, this salad contains macro and micronutrients that are beneficial for hormone health, including the omega-3s in the flaxseed and lemon dressing. This delicious mix of flavors will keep your appetite, your hormones, and your blood sugar levels stable and satisfied for hours.

2 cups (56g) shredded red leaf lettuce

1 cup (70g) shredded red cabbage

1 pound (455g) cooked chicken breast, turkey, fish, or shrimp, chopped

½ of a red bell pepper, cut julienne

1 cup (130g) jicama, cut julienne

1 small avocado, peeled and diced

¼ cup (60g) canned black beans, drained and rinsed

¼ of a red onion, thinly sliced

¼ cup (35g) pumpkin seeds

¼ cup (60ml) flaxseed oil

2 to 3 tablespoons fresh lemon or lime juice

Dash of cayenne pepper

Freshly ground black pepper

▶ *Combine the lettuce and next 8 ingredients (through pumpkin seeds) in a large serving bowl. Whisk together the flaxseed oil, lemon juice, cayenne pepper, and black pepper. Toss with the salad.*

Yield: *4 servings*

Each with: Calories 885.17; Calories From Fat 442.36; Total Fat 50.64g; Cholesterol 192.78mg; Sodium 342.86mg; Potassium 1549.25mg; Total Carbohydrates 30.77g; Fiber 13.38g; Sugar 3.59g; Protein 77.77g

Health Facilitators	Nutrient Density Rating	Blood Sugar Balance Rating
Protein	High	
Fat	High	
Carbohydrate	High	Very High
Enzymes	High	
Antioxidants	High	
Fiber	High	

BLOOD SUGAR–STABILIZING SESAME-COCONUT CRUSTED SALMON

Enjoy the nutty flavor of this delicious salmon coated with calcium-rich sesame seeds. Coconuts contain both lauric and caprylic acid, which are soothing as well as antimicrobial and antifungal. And the omega-3s in the salmon benefit your hormones and your blood sugar levels.

1 tablespoon (20g) maple syrup

¼ cup (60ml) purified water

¼ cup (60ml) tamari sauce (wheat-free) or Bragg's liquid amino acids

1 tablespoon (6g) peeled, chopped fresh ginger

1 garlic clove, chopped

4 salmon steaks, about 3 to 4 ounces (85 to 115g) each

3 tablespoons (21g) coconut flour

¼ cup (26g) sesame seeds

2 tablespoons (11g) desiccated coconut

2 tablespoons (28g) coconut oil

2 tablespoons (28ml) sesame oil

4 cups (120g) spinach, steamed

▶ *Combine the maple syrup, tamari, ginger, and garlic in a bowl. Add the salmon steaks to the bowl and marinate for 45 minutes or overnight in the refrigerator. In a resealable plastic bag, combine the flour with sesame seeds and desiccated coconut. Drop the marinated fish into the bag and coat with the flour and seeds. Heat the coconut and sesame oils in a frying pan over medium-high heat. Sauté the salmon steaks for 2 to 3 minutes on each side or to the desired doneness. Serve over steamed spinach.*

Yield: *4 servings*

Each with: Calories 426.4; Calories From Fat 273.52; Total Fat 31.17g; Cholesterol 61mg; Sodium 1086.3mg; Potassium 645.62mg; Total Carbohydrates 13.83g; Fiber 4.39g; Sugar 4.32g; Protein 25.49g

Health Facilitators	Nutrient Density Rating	Blood Sugar Balance Rating
Protein	High	
Fat	High	
Carbohydrate	Medium	Very High
Enzymes	Low	
Antioxidants	High	
Fiber	Medium	

COMFORTING QUINOA-CRAB CASSEROLE

Having a busy night? Try this easy dish that's high in calcium, magnesium, and selenium to calm you while keeping your blood sugar levels stable. Quinoa is a nutrient-dense grain that contains nearly twice the amount of protein per cup (225 g) found in other grains. Pair this recipe with a side of tossed greens and a medley of your favorite veggies for extra nutrients.

½ pound (225g) cooked crabmeat

2 celery stalks, finely chopped

1 red bell pepper, diced

⅓ cup (33g) chopped black olives

¼ cup (4g) finely chopped cilantro

1 medium brown or red onion, finely chopped

2 large garlic cloves, minced

1 teaspoon fresh basil, chopped

1 teaspoon fresh oregano, chopped

Salt and pepper

Dash of cayenne pepper

1 egg

1 cup (185g) cooked quinoa

1 cup (230g) plain yogurt

Juice of ½ of a lemon

1 tablespoon (15ml) extra-virgin olive oil or coconut
   oil (melted)

▶ Preheat the oven to 350°F (180°C, or gas mark 4). Mix the crab, celery, red bell pepper, olives, cilantro, onion, garlic, basil, oregano, salt, pepper, and cayenne pepper in a bowl. Whisk the egg in a separate bowl and blend with the quinoa, yogurt, and lemon juice. Gradually stir the egg mixture into the crab mixture. Place in a lightly oiled 10-inch (25 cm) casserole dish. Bake for 15 to 20 minutes.

Yield: *4 servings*

Each with: Calories 248.96; Calories From Fat 74.95;
Total Fat 8.56g; Cholesterol 99.64mg; Sodium 397.94mg;
Potassium 685.1mg; Total Carbohydrates 22.55g; Fiber 3.55g;
Sugar 7.84g; Protein 20.61g

Health Facilitators	Nutrient Density Rating	Blood Sugar Balance Rating
Protein	High	
Fat	Medium	
Carbohydrate	Medium	Very High
Enzymes	Low	
Antioxidants	High	
Fiber	High	

MOOD-BOOSTING MEATLOAF WITH A KICK

This is real comfort food that is not only great for your hormones but for your blood sugar levels too. It's loaded with protein and calming tryptophan and has a deliciously sweet and spicy kick thanks to the raisins and herbs like garlic (a great antioxidant). This dish is delightfully easy and simple to prepare and goes straight into the oven for an hour after the prep work is complete. It tastes great as leftovers, for breakfast, lunch, or dinner, or even as a quick snack. Serve it with a salad or steamed vegetables to round out the meal.

1 to 2 tablespoons (15 to 28ml) extra-virgin olive oil or coconut oil (melted)

2 pounds (900g) ground turkey

1 cup (185g) cooked quinoa

¾ cup (120g) chopped brown or red onion

2 cloves of garlic, chopped

2 tablespoons (30g) horseradish

2 tablespoons (2g) chopped cilantro

2 tablespoons (8g) chopped parsley

½ cup (75g) raisins

1 teaspoon salt (optional)

¼ teaspoon pepper

1 teaspoon dry mustard

1 teaspoon cumin powder

½ cup (120g) ketchup

2 eggs, lightly beaten

▶ Preheat the oven to 350°F (180°C, or gas mark 4). Coat an 8 x 4 x 2-inch (20 x 10 x 5 cm) glass loaf pan with olive oil. Combine the remaining ingredients, blending by hand to mix thoroughly. Shape the mixture and place in the prepared loaf pan. Bake for 1 hour.

Yield: *5 to 6 servings*

Each with: Calories 381.92; Calories From Fat 155.75; Total Fat 17.34g; Cholesterol 189.95mg; Sodium 798.44mg; Potassium 677.55mg; Total Carbohydrates 25.79g; Fiber 2.11g; Sugar 14.1g; Protein 31.18g 62%

Health Facilitators	Nutrient Density Rating	Blood Sugar Balance Rating
Protein	High	
Fat	High	
Carbohydrate	Medium	Very High
Enzymes	Low	
Antioxidants	High	
Fiber	High	

COLONIAL BAKED APPLES WITH CHERRIES

Easy is the operative word here. This dessert is easy to make—and even easier to eat. Try these cherry and nut filled baked apples for breakfast, brunch, or dessert. Cherries are low on the glycemic index and contain an abundance of antioxidants, such as vitamin C. Apples are also high in vitamin C, which stabilizes blood sugar levels and minimizes sugar cravings.

2 tablespoons (28 ml) freshly squeezed lemon juice

⅓ cup (53g) dried cherries

3 tablespoons (24g) chopped walnuts

1 teaspoon grated lemon zest

2 tablespoons (40g) honey or maple syrup

6 apples, cored

▶ Preheat the oven to 350°F (180°C, or gas mark 4). Spray a baking sheet with nonstick vegetable spray. In a bowl, mix together the lemon juice, cherries, walnuts, lemon zest, and honey or maple syrup. Place the cored apples on the baking sheet. Fill each apple with the cherry-nut mixture. Bake until the apples are soft, about 30 to 40 minutes.

Yield: *6 servings*

Each with: Calories 141.75: Calories From Fat 23.45; Total Fat 2.8g; Cholesterol 0mg; Sodium 3.23mg; Potassium 184.63mg; Total Carbohydrates 31.19g; Fiber 4.06g; Sugar 18.54g; Protein 1.17g

Health Facilitators	Nutrient Density Rating	Blood Sugar Balance Rating
Protein	Medium	
Fat	Medium	
Carbohydrate	High	Medium
Enzymes	Low	
Antioxidants	Medium	
Fiber	High	

RECIPES FOR
ALL SUGAR ADDICTION TYPES

The healing properties in the recipes in this section make them suitable for all four types of sugar addicts. Supplying your body with essential nutrients is your best bet for keeping your blood sugar levels stable and weaning yourself off sugar. In fact, when you start eating these low-sugar, healthful recipes, you will be surprised at how quickly you lose your interest in sweets. Most people are freed from their sugar cravings in a relatively short amount of time—just a few days! Start by using the recipes for your specific type(s) and add in these recipes once you start to feel better. After a few months, you'll be amazed at how balanced your blood sugar is and how good you feel. You are healing your sugar addiction bite by bite!

BERRY-NUTTY SMOOTHIE

High in vitamin C (one serving contains 14 mg, or 25 percent of your daily requirement), fiber, manganese, and antioxidant power, the tiny blueberry is one of the healthiest fruits around. Strawberries also contain vitamin C, along with folic acid, potassium, and fiber. Protein powder, rich peanut or almond butter, and yogurt make this smoothie a balancing meal or snack and a favorite you'll make again and again.

1 cup (155g) frozen blueberries

¼ cup (64g) frozen strawberries

4 to 6 tablespoons (60 to 90g) plain yogurt

2 tablespoons (28ml) flax oil

2 to 4 tablespoons (32 to 64g) crunchy peanut butter or almond butter

2 to 4 scoops (⅔ to 1⅓ cups, or 107 to 213g) protein powder

1¾ cups (410ml) purified water

1 cup (235ml) ice (optional)

▶ Place all the ingredients in a blender. Blend until rich and creamy, approximately 2 to 3 minutes.

Yield: *2 servings*

Each with: Calories 497.19; Calories From Fat; Total Fat 32.58g; Cholesterol 1.84mg; Sodium 252.51mg; Potassium 394.87mg; Total Carbohydrates 26.01g; Fiber 7.23g; Sugar 14.66g; Protein 36.75g

Health Facilitators	Nutrient Density Rating	Blood Sugar Balance Rating
Protein	High	
Fat	High	
Carbohydrate	Medium	High
Enzymes	High	
Antioxidants	Very High	
Fiber	Medium	

STABILIZING EGGS SUPREME

You'll feel full for hours after you eat this delicious, blood sugar–stabilizing dish that provides protein and good fats and contains vitamins A, D, B$_{12}$, and riboflavin for strengthening your immune system. Switch out the dairy for tofu if you're lactose intolerant, and you won't miss a nutritional thing.

4 eggs

2 tablespoons (28ml) heavy cream

Freshly ground black pepper

Dash of cayenne pepper

1 tablespoon (15ml) extra-virgin olive oil or coconut oil (melted)

1 small red onion, chopped

1 garlic clove, minced

1 tablespoon (14g) unsalted butter

3 tablespoons (45g) cream cheese, cut into small cubes

1 sliced ripe avocado

2 cups (60g) spinach or (110g) mixed salad greens

▶ Preheat the broiler. In a medium bowl, using a fork, whisk the eggs, cream, black pepper, and cayenne pepper. Set the mixture aside. In a nonstick skillet, melt the oil over medium-high heat. When the oil is hot, sauté the onions and garlic until the onions are translucent, about 5 minutes. Remove from the skillet and set aside.

Melt the butter in the skillet and add the egg mixture. As the eggs cook, lift the edges to allow any uncooked egg to seep underneath. When the bottom is set but the top is still moist, place the cream cheese cubes and onion mixture over the eggs and place under the broiler. Broil 1 to 2 minutes, checking frequently, until the top is golden and puffed up. Top with sliced avocado. Serve over a bed of spinach or salad greens

Yield: *2 to 3 servings*

Each with: Calories 369.96; Calories From Fat 285.36; Total Fat 32.8g; Cholesterol 321.83mg; Sodium 162.27mg; Potassium 524.41mg; Total Carbohydrates 10.41g; Fiber 5.05g; Sugar 0.83g; Protein 11.92g

Health Facilitators	Nutrient Density Rating	Blood Sugar Balance Rating
Protein	High	
Fat	High	
Carbohydrate	Medium	Very High
Enzymes	Low	
Antioxidants	High	
Fiber	Low	

BLOOD SUGAR–BALANCING BUCKWHEAT BREAD

This nutritious loaf is a fabulous golden yellow, and the texture reminds you of how bread should taste: filling and delicious. Slice it thinly and add your favorite low-glycemic toppings (such as avocado, hummus, or mashed bananas) for extra nutrient density and to increase blood sugar balance. This bread is a great accompaniment to soups and salads too. It is gluten-, dairy-, and wheat-free and will keep for up to three days.

1¼ cups (150g) buckwheat pancake mix

1 cup (140g) polenta or maize meal

2 teaspoons baking powder

1 teaspoon salt

1 egg

1 cup (235ml) coconut or rice milk

⅓ cup (80ml) purified water

¼ cup (60ml) extra-virgin olive oil, plus more for pan

▶ *Preheat the oven to 350°F (180°C, or gas mark 4). Brush an 8-inch (20 cm) loaf pan with olive oil, line with parchment paper, and also brush the parchment paper with oil. Place the pancake mix, polenta, baking powder, and salt in a large bowl and combine thoroughly. In a small bowl, beat the egg and add the coconut or rice milk, water, and oil. Add the egg mixture to the dry ingredients and stir until well blended. Pour into the prepared loaf pan and bake for 30 minutes. Rotate the pan and bake for another 12 to 15 minutes. It is done when a skewer comes out clean. Remove from the pan immediately and peel off the paper lining. Cool on a wire rack in fresh air to develop a crust. It is best served the same day or toasted over the next couple of days.*

Yield: *6 to 8 servings*

Amount Per Serving; Calories 314.37; Calories From Fat 122.40; Total Fat 14.16g; Cholesterol 26.44mg; Sodium 689.84mg; Potassium 131.22mg; Total Carbohydrates 41.68g; Fiber 5.11g; Sugar 1.42g; Protein 6.42g

Health Facilitators	Nutrient Density Rating	Blood Sugar Balance Rating
Protein	Medium	
Fat	Medium	
Carbohydrate	High	High
Enzymes	Low	
Antioxidants	Low	
Fiber	High	

STRENGTHENING MINESTRONE

Minestrone is the "everything but the kitchen sink" of soups and is a nourishing and satisfying dish for all of the four types. A little of this and a little of that add up to a quick and easy Italian classic. The combination of vitamins and minerals are strengthening and boost immune function. Feel free to add your favorite meat or some lentils for added protein. A sprinkling of freshly grated Parmesan cheese is a wonderful finishing touch and a calcium-rich blood sugar–balancer.

1 tablespoon (15ml) extra-virgin olive oil

4 medium cloves of garlic, minced

1 small onion, diced

2 medium stalks of celery, diced

2 medium carrots, cut into ½-inch (1.3cm) slices

¼ teaspoon finely chopped thyme

¼ teaspoon finely chopped parsley

⅛ teaspoon black pepper

⅛ teaspoon salt

3 cups (700ml) vegetable stock, divided

½ cup (90g) canned diced tomatoes, drained

½ cup (35g) shredded savoy cabbage

3 cups (700ml) vegetable juice

½ cup (89g) cooked red kidney beans

½ cup (93g) brown rice

▶ In a soup pot, heat the oil over medium heat and sauté the garlic and onion until the onion is translucent, about 5 minutes. Add the celery, carrots, thyme, parsley, black pepper, and salt. Moisten with 3 tablespoons (45 ml) of the stock and cook for 5 minutes. Add the tomatoes, cabbage, vegetable juice, and remaining stock and bring to a boil. Lower the heat, stir in the beans and brown rice, and simmer, covered, for 20 to 30 minutes.

Yield: *8 servings*

Each with: Calories 143.81; Calories From Fat 29.63; Total Fat 3.34g; Cholesterol 2.7mg; Sodium 426.73mg; Potassium 567.6mg; Total Carbohydrates 24.62g; Fiber 3.76g; Sugar 6.46g; Protein 5.38g

Health Facilitators	Nutrient Density Rating	Blood Sugar Balance Rating
Protein	Medium	
Fat	Medium	
Carbohydrate	High	High
Enzymes	Low	
Antioxidants	High	
Fiber	High	

TRYPTOPHAN-RICH TURMERIC TURKEY BURGERS

Turkey is not only low in fat and good for your waistline, but it is also high in tryptophan, which will keep your mood and your blood sugar levels stable. It's also highly nutritious, with selenium and B vitamins, as well as zinc, making it ideal for keeping your immune system strong. The health benefits of curcumin, the active ingredient in turmeric, are well documented. Not only does it contain numerous antioxidants, it is also anti-inflammatory and improves digestion, circulation, and energy. It may even help in fat metabolism and weight management and prevent premature aging.

1 pound (455g) ground turkey

1 teaspoon turmeric

1 teaspoon cumin

½ red or brown onion, chopped

1 clove of garlic, finely chopped

¼ cup (4g) chopped cilantro

¼ cup (15g) chopped parsley

¼ teaspoon salt

Black pepper

Dash of cayenne pepper

1 egg, beaten

2 tablespoons (28ml) extra-virgin olive oil or coconut oil (melted)

3 cups (165g) mixed greens or (60g) spinach

▶ Mix the first 11 ingredients (through the egg) in a bowl. Form this mixture into four patties. Heat the oil in a skillet over medium heat, add the patties, and sauté until cooked through and no longer pink, about 7 to 10 minutes. Serve over a bed of mixed salad or spinach greens.

Yield: *4 servings*

Each with: Calories 265.01; Calories From Fat 158.05; Total Fat 17.69g; Cholesterol 142.46mg; Sodium 292.84mg; Potassium 491.56mg; Total Carbohydrates 3.57g; Fiber 1.16g; Sugar 0.91g; Protein 22.54g

Health Facilitators	Nutrient Density Rating	Blood Sugar Balance Rating
Protein	Very High	
Fat	Low	
Carbohydrate	Low	Very High
Enzymes	Low	
Antioxidants	High	
Fiber	Low	

SUPERCHARGED CHICKEN AND GREENS

Enjoy the delicious flavors and textures in the nutrient-dense and blood sugar–stabilizing salad. Perfect for all four sugar addiction types, it contains just the right amount of protein plus omega-3 essential fatty acids (from the nuts). The vegetables and herbs add a nice zing and are full of antioxidants for greater energy, making you less likely to reach for sugar to pep you up!

1½ pounds (680g) cooked chicken breast, cubed or stripped

1 cup (100g) chopped scallions

¾ cup (75g) chopped celery

1 cup (100g) green beans, raw or lightly steamed

2 tablespoons (16g) golden sesame seeds

Salt and pepper

¼ cup (60ml) extra-virgin olive oil or coconut oil (melted)

2 tablespoons (28ml) fresh lemon or lime juice

1 tablespoon (15g) Dijon mustard

2 tablespoons (28ml) purified water

6 cups (216g) chopped green leaf lettuce

6 walnuts or macadamia nuts, chopped

▶ Mix the chicken, scallions, celery, green beans, and sesame seeds in a large bowl. Season with salt and pepper to taste. In a separate bowl, make the vinaigrette by whisking the oil, lemon or lime juice, Dijon mustard, and water together. Toss the greens and vinaigrette in a large bowl; arrange a single serving on each plate. Top each serving with the chicken mixture and a sprinkling of chopped nuts.

Yield: *6 servings*

Each with: Calories 340.98; Calories From Fat 157.37; Total Fat 17.98g; Cholesterol 96.39mg; Sodium 136.33mg; Potassium 598.49mg; Total Carbohydrates 6.79g; Fiber 3.25g; Sugar 1.85g; Protein 38g

Health Facilitators	Nutrient Density Rating	Blood Sugar Balance Rating
Protein	High	
Fat	Medium	
Carbohydrate	Medium	Very High
Enzymes	High	
Antioxidants	High	
Fiber	High	

ANTIOXIDANT-RICH RATATOUILLE

The vegetables in this dish are loaded with antioxidants, vitamins B and C, numerous minerals, and tons of fiber. The antioxidants protect brain cells as well as strengthen your immune system. And the oil adds healthy fats to keep blood sugar levels stable.

3 tablespoons (45ml) extra-virgin olive oil or coconut oil (melted)

1 large onion, chopped

3 minced garlic cloves

1 large eggplant, (peeled, if desired) and cut into ½-inch (1.3cm) cubes

1 red bell pepper, cut into ½-inch (1.3cm) pieces

1 green bell pepper, cut into ½-inch (1.3cm) pieces

1 large zucchini, cut into ¼-inch (0.6cm) half circles

1 cup (100g) green beans, ends trimmed, and sliced diagonally into 1-inch (2.5cm) pieces

6 large ripe tomatoes, chopped

2 tablespoons (32g) tomato paste

¼ cup (15g) chopped fresh parsley

¼ cup (60ml) red wine

½ cup (120ml) water

2 tablespoons (5g) slivered fresh basil, or 2 teaspoons dried basil

½ teaspoon dried thyme

½ teaspoon dried rosemary

½ teaspoon dried marjoram

1 bay leaf

1 tablespoon (15ml) balsamic vinegar

Finely ground black pepper

▶ In a large Dutch oven, heat the oil over medium-high heat. When the oil is hot, add the onion and garlic and sauté until softened, about 5 minutes. Add the eggplant and bell peppers and cook until softened, about 8 minutes more. Add the zucchini and next 11 ingredients (through the bay leaf). Mix well. Bring to a boil. Reduce the heat and simmer, uncovered, 20 minutes, stirring occasionally. Add the balsamic vinegar and black pepper. Taste and adjust the seasonings. Simmer another 15 minutes. Remove the bay leaf and discard. Serve hot, warm, or cold.

Yield: *4 to 6 servings*

Each with: Calories 154.07; Calories From Fat 65.75; Total Fat 7.47g; Cholesterol 0mg; Sodium 62.12mg; Potassium 856.52mg; Total Carbohydrates 19.41g; Fiber 7.09g; Sugar 9.83g; Protein 3.89g

Health Facilitators	Nutrient Density Rating	Blood Sugar Balance Rating
Protein	Medium	
Fat	Low	
Carbohydrate	High	High
Enzymes	High	
Antioxidants	High	
Fiber	High	

SIMPLE ROAST CHICKEN WITH HEALING HERBS

Ideal for all four sugar addiction types, this dish is simple, easy, delicious, and nutritious. High in tryptophan and protein, it keeps you looking on the bright side and off the sugar roller coaster. Leftovers are wonderful for lunch the next day!

1 head of garlic, cut in half

2 lemons, sliced in thirds

1 bunch of rosemary

1 bunch of marjoram

1 (3½- to 4-pound, or 1.6 to 1.8kg) chicken, 4 bone-in chicken breasts, or 1 large turkey breast

½ cup (120ml) purified water

2 tablespoons (28ml) extra-virgin olive oil

▶ Preheat the oven to 350°F (180°C, or gas mark 4). If using a whole chicken, discard the giblets and rinse and pat dry. Place the chicken on a roasting pan and stuff the cavity with the garlic, lemon pieces, rosemary, and marjoram. If using the chicken or turkey breasts, in a shallow baking dish, scatter the garlic, lemons, and herbs evenly across the bottom. Place the chicken or turkey on top. Add the water to the pan and baste the chicken or turkey with the oil. Bake until the juices run clear when pierced with a fork, about 1½ to 2 hours for the whole chicken, or until the internal temperature reaches 160°F (71°C), or about 30 minutes for chicken or turkey breasts.

Yield: *4 servings*

Amount Per Serving; Calories 123.8; Calories From Fat 62.89; Total Fat 7.22g; Cholesterol 15.12mg; Sodium 460.88mg; Potassium 166.77mg; Total Carbohydrates 11.09g; Fiber 3.08g; Sugar 0.18g; Protein 8.54g

Health Facilitators	Nutrient Density Rating	Blood Sugar Balance Rating
Protein	High	
Fat	Medium	
Carbohydrate	Low	Very High
Enzymes	Low	
Antioxidants	Low	
Fiber	Low	

HIGH-ENERGY GARLIC SHRIMP

Low-calorie, high-protein shrimp are rich in B vitamins, contain iodine to support your thyroid naturally, and their protein make them a go-to choice for stabilizing blood sugar levels. It is also a good source of magnesium, which studies suggest can help prevent type 2 diabetes. Serve with a large mixed green salad.

For the Spicy Garlic Sauce:

2 to 3 garlic cloves, peeled and minced

1 cup (235ml) plus 3 tablespoons (45ml)
  purified water, divided

⅓ cup (80ml) toasted sesame oil

1 tablespoon (15ml) hot pepper sauce

1 tablespoon (20g) maple syrup

3 tablespoons (45ml) shoyu

1 teaspoon red pepper flakes

1 tablespoon (8g) kudzu or arrowroot starch

For the Shrimp:

¼ cup (60ml) purified water

½ teaspoon coconut oil

1 red or brown onion, sliced thinly

1 bunch of broccoli, florets and stems separated
  (cut stems into thin rounds)

1 carrot, sliced thinly on the diagonal

1 pound (455g) wild-caught shrimp,
  peeled and deveined

▶ *To make the garlic sauce: Mix all the ingredients except for the kudzu and 3 tablespoons (45ml) water in a small saucepan and cook over medium heat for 3 minutes. Dilute the kudzu in 3 tablespoons (45ml) water and slowly add to the pan. The sauce will begin to thicken. Cook for 3 to 5 minutes or until the kudzu becomes clear.*

To make the shrimp: Add the water, oil, and onion to a frying pan and cook over medium heat for 1 to 2 minutes. Add the broccoli stems and carrot and cook for 2 minutes. Add the broccoli florets and shrimp, cover the pan, and steam for 2 to 3 minutes. Add the Spicy Garlic Sauce to the pan. Cover and cook over medium heat for another 5 minutes.

Yield: *2 to 4 servings*

Each with: Calories 369.6; Calories From Fat 215.07; Total Fat 24.32g; Cholesterol 172.37mg; Sodium 873.85mg; Potassium 500.23mg; Total Carbohydrates 12.81g; Fiber 1.21g; Sugar 5.45g; Protein 25.67g

Health Facilitators	Nutrient Density Rating	Blood Sugar Balance Rating
Protein	High	
Fat	High	
Carbohydrate	Low	Very High
Enzymes	Low	
Antioxidants	Medium	
Fiber	Low	

TRANSFORMING TEMPEH

Tempeh is an excellent choice for all four types who have difficulty digesting plant-based high-protein foods like beans and legumes or soy foods such as tofu. That's because the process of fermentation makes the soybeans softer and easier to digest. High in calcium, zinc, and iron, along with the dozens of antioxidants from the vegetables, this dish is packed with nutrients to keep blood sugar levels stable. Serve over steamed brown rice.

3 tablespoons (45ml) peanut oil or (45g) coconut oil

3 cloves of garlic, finely chopped or minced

½ of a red onion, chopped

1 tablespoon (6g) fresh ginger, peeled and finely chopped

½ teaspoon red pepper flakes

4 medium zucchini, cut into ¼-inch (6mm) circles

2 red bell peppers, slivered

1 pound (455g) tempeh, cut into ½-inch (1.3cm) squares

2 tablespoons (28ml) tamari sauce (wheat-free), or Bragg's liquid amino acids

2 tablespoons (28ml) sesame oil

1 tablespoon (15ml) fresh lime juice

2 tablespoons (12g) chopped scallions,

2 tablespoons (2g) chopped fresh cilantro

▶ *In a wok or a large nonstick skillet, heat the peanut oil over medium to high heat. When the oil is hot, add the garlic, onions, and ginger and cook for 30 seconds, stirring constantly. Add the red pepper flakes, zucchini, red bell pepper, and tempeh and stir-fry about 7 minutes until the vegetables are tender. In a separate bowl, combine the tamari or Bragg's liquid amino acid, sesame oil, lime juice, scallions, and cilantro. Pour over the tempeh and vegetables and cook, stirring, until heated through. Taste and adjust the seasonings.*

Yield: *4 servings*

Each with: Calories 441.66; Calories From Fat 257.78; Total Fat 29.84g; Cholesterol 0mg; Sodium 539.32mg; Potassium 1220.25mg; Total Carbohydrates 25.28g; Fiber 4.35g; Sugar 6.95g; Protein 25.63g

Health Facilitators	Nutrient Density Rating	Blood Sugar Balance Rating
Protein	High	
Fat	Medium	
Carbohydrate	Medium	Very High
Enzymes	Medium	
Antioxidants	High	
Fiber	High	

SPICE-IT-UP SAUSAGES WITH LENTILS AND LEEKS

Leeks are a small but mighty member of the onion family. Packed with plant protein, rich in vitamins C, B$_6$, and folate, plus iron and manganese, leeks balance blood sugar and even raise HDL or "good" cholesterol. Leeks are particularly high in tryptophan, which means mellow moods and a good night's sleep. Combined with tasty sausage, fresh herbs, and garlic, this dish is a go-to meal for all four types. Enjoy this one for lunch or dinner or as a hearty snack, served with brown rice.

2 tablespoons (28ml) olive oil

½ of a brown onion, chopped

2 garlic cloves, peeled and minced

1 large leek, cleaned and chopped

2 cups (60g) spinach, cleaned and chopped

2 tablespoons (4g) fresh thyme

2 tablespoons (2g) chopped cilantro

2 cups (384g) dried lentils, soaked overnight

3½ cups (820ml) purified water

2 bay leaves

1½ pounds (680g) chicken sausage links
(or pork, turkey, or tofu), diced

1 teaspoon sea salt

Freshly ground black pepper

Dash of cayenne pepper

▶ Heat the oil in a large skillet over medium-high heat. Sauté the onion, garlic, and leek 1 to 2 minutes. Add the spinach and cook until wilted, about 3 to 5 minutes. Add the thyme, cilantro, lentils (discard lentil soaking water), purified water, and bay leaves. Bring to a boil, cover, and simmer over low heat for 30 minutes. Add the diced sausage, salt, black pepper, and cayenne pepper. Continue cooking for another 30 minutes or until the lentils are soft.

Yield: *4 to 6 servings*

Each with: Calories 331.44; Calories From Fat 70.4;
Total Fat 7.8g; Cholesterol 18.75mg; Sodium 528.8mg;
Potassium 727.26mg; Total Carbohydrates 42.74g;
Fiber 20.62g; Sugar 2.36g; Protein 22.78g

Health Facilitators	Nutrient Density Rating	Blood Sugar Balance Rating
Protein	High	
Fat	Medium	
Carbohydrate	High	Very High
Enzymes	Low	
Antioxidants	Medium	
Fiber	High	

NOURISHING APPLE NUT CAKE

The combination of the healthy fat in coconuts (lauric acid), the high fiber and antioxidants in apples, and heart-healthy walnuts means this dessert is nourishing and blood sugar–balancing. The orange juice makes this cake moist and delicious. You're sure to want more of this tasty treat!

4 large apples, cored, peeled, and sliced

2 tablespoons (15g) chopped walnuts

4 teaspoons (8g) cinnamon

6 dates, chopped

1 cup (145g) raisins

3 cups (336g) coconut flour

1 tablespoon (14g) baking powder

½ cup (120ml) coconut oil (melted)

4 large eggs

½ cup (120ml) freshly squeezed orange juice

1 tablespoon (15ml) melted butter

▶ Preheat the oven to 350°F (180°C, or gas mark 4). Grease a 10-inch (25 cm) tube pan or loaf pan. In a medium bowl, blend the apples, walnuts, cinnamon, dates, and raisins. In a separate bowl, combine the flour, baking powder, oil, eggs, orange juice, and butter. Beat 4 to 5 minutes with an electric mixer until the batter is smooth. Pour half of the batter into the pan and spread half of the apple mixture on top. Repeat the procedure and bake for 30 minutes. Then lower the oven temperature to 300°F (150°C, or gas mark 2) and bake for another hour or until a toothpick inserted into the center comes out clean.

Yield: *4 to 6 servings*

Each with: Calories 645.8; Calories From Fat 272.81; Total Fat 31.41g; Cholesterol 146.09mg; Sodium 308.64mg; Potassium 464.39mg; Total Carbohydrates 85.49g; Fiber 29.02g; Sugar 33.19g; Protein 14.09g

Health Facilitators	Nutrient Density Rating	Blood Sugar Balance Rating
Protein	Medium	
Fat	High	
Carbohydrate	High	High
Enzymes	Low	
Antioxidants	Medium	
Fiber	High	

FRESH STRAWBERRIES CHANTILLY GONE NUTS

The sweet juiciness and deep red color of strawberries can brighten up both the flavor and look of any meal. Strawberries are loaded with antioxidants, especially vitamin C, which protect against harmful free radicals. The tasty fruit is also high in fiber, potassium, and iodine, which makes them effective at boosting thyroid function. The walnuts add omega-3 essential fatty acids, and the delicious healthy fats in crème fraîche help stabilize your blood sugar levels. This dish makes a perfect snack or sweet ending to a meal!

8 cups (1.4kg) fresh strawberries, washed, dried, hulled, and quartered

¼ cup (45g) chopped dates

¼ cup (60ml) freshly squeezed orange juice

1½ cups (345g) crème fraîche

3 to 4 tablespoons (24 to 32g) walnuts, chopped

8 mint sprigs

▶ Divide the strawberries among 8 serving bowls. In a mixing bowl, combine the chopped dates, orange juice, and the crème fraîche and mix well. Place 3 tablespoons (45g) of the date mixture on top of each serving of strawberries and garnish with walnuts and a sprig of mint.

If these recipes have whet your appetite for more healthy dishes, check out *The Beat Sugar Addiction Now Cookbook!* (Fair Winds Press, 2011). Bon Appetite!

Yield: *8 servings*

Each with: Calories 214.96; Calories From Fat 20.07; Total Fat 13.11g; Cholesterol 26.89mg; Sodium 2.32mg; Potassium 383.95mg; Total Carbohydrates 23.42g; Fiber 4.74g; Sugar 15.5g; Protein 2.83g

Health Facilitators	Nutrient Density Rating	Blood Sugar Balance Rating
Protein	Low	
Fat	High	
Carbohydrate	High	High
Enzymes	High	
Antioxidants	High	
Fiber	High	

APPENDIX A

TREATMENT PLANS SIMPLIFIED

In this appendix, you'll find information about many combination products that can simplify your treatment plan, along with specific brands we recommend. Unless noted, the natural supplements suggested here can be found in most health food stores, at www.endfatigue.com (or by calling [800] 333-5287), or at most online natural pharmacies. I consider Enzymatic Therapy (sold in health food stores) and Integrative Therapeutics and Europharma (sold to health care practitioners) to be two of the best brands.

In appendix D, you'll find the addresses, phone numbers, and websites for the companies who make and/or distribute the products recommended here. You'll also find information about compounding pharmacies, finding the best water filter, and more.

When taking the supplements that are right for your individual condition and/or sugar addiction type, I usually suggest the following:

- Begin to slowly taper off most treatments when you have felt well for six months. I recommend the vitamin powder (treatment #1, below) for long-term use to maintain optimal nutritional support.

- Stop supplements one at a time, so you can see whether you still need them.

- If need be, any or all of these can be used forever, although this is usually not necessary.

I encourage people who recommend either prescription or natural products to provide financial disclosure of financial ties they may have to the makers of the products they recommend. A word about Fatigued to Fantastic products: I direct any company making my formulas to donate to charity all of the money that I would have received. I also never accept money from any natural or pharmaceutical product companies. I do make money from products sold on my website (www.endfatigue.com).

Note that most of the supplements recommended below can be found at your local health food store or at www.endfatigue.com.

OPTIMAL OVERALL NUTRITIONAL SUPPORT FOR ALL SUGAR ADDICTS

☐ **1. Energy Revitalization System multivitamin powder (Berry or Citrus by Enzymatic Therapy):** Take one-half to one scoop a day (as feels best) blended with milk, water, or yogurt. If diarrhea occurs, mix the powder with milk and/or start with a lower dose and work your way up to the dose that feels best; or, divide the daily dose into smaller doses and take two or three times a day. It's available at www.endfatigue.com and most health food stores.

Supplements for Type 1 Sugar Addiction

To Increase Energy

☐ **2. Ribose (by Bioenergy):** Take one 5-gram scoop of powder three times a day for three weeks, then twice a day. If this is too energizing, take it with food or lower the dose. The effects are usually seen within two to three weeks. You can find it at your health food store or at www.endfatigue.com.

To Treat Insomnia

☐ **3. Revitalizing Sleep Formula (from Enzymatic Therapies or Integrative Therapeutics):** This formula contains 200 mg of valerian, 90 mg of passionflower, 50 mg of L-theanine, 30 mg of hops, 20 mg of lemon balm, and 28 mg of wild lettuce. Take two to four capsules each night up to sixty minutes before bedtime. It can also be used during the day for anxiety. If valerian energizes you (this occurs in 5 to 10 percent of people), use the other components. Do not take more than eight capsules a day.

Magnesium and More

☐ **4. Sustained-Release Magnesium (by Jigsaw Health):** If taking magnesium causes diarrhea, use this form (it contains 125 mg per tablet, plus other helpful nutrients).

☐ **4a. Calm Aid:** This is a new supplement that contains lavender essential oil, called Silexan, and is clinically proven to help if you have insomnia. Take it at bedtime. When combined with other sleep aids, this makes them more effective. You'll find it at most drugstores and online merchants.

Supplements for Type 2 Sugar Addiction

For Adrenal Support

☐ **5. Adrenal Stress End (from Enzymatic Therapies or Integrative Therapeutics):** This combination product contains important nutrients for adrenal health. Take one or two capsules each morning (or one or two in the morning and another at noon). Lower the dosage or take with food if it upsets your stomach (which is unusual).

Supplements for Type 3 Sugar Addiction

To Promote Healthy Gut Flora

☐ **6. Berberine:** Take between 250–500 mg three times a day for gut infections (less if you've got an upset stomach).

☐ **7. Acidophilus Milk Bacteria, Acidophilus Pearls, Probiotic Pearls, and Pearls Elite (from Enzymatic Therapy or Integrative Therapeutics):** Take one Pearls Elite for five months and then consider taking one every other day to help maintain healthy bowels. The Enzymatic Therapy contain about 5 billion units per pearl. I use only probiotics made in protective "pearls"; otherwise, your stomach acid will kill 99.9 percent of the bacteria, making them useless for fighting yeast. For gut "intensive care," begin with one 50 billion unit Optima Digestive Balance capsule daily for one month.

☐ **7a. Lauricidin (Monolaurin):** Take it with or after meals. The mini pellets can be placed in the mouth and swallowed with water. Don't chew or take with hot liquids or it will taste oily. You may experience a die off reaction, so go slow and start with 750 mg (1/4 of the blue scoop) or less one to two times daily for a week before increasing the amount. The level can then be increased to 1.5 grams (1/2 of the blue scoop) one to two times a day. One container is enough to tell if it will help you.

Supplements for Type 4 Sugar Addiction

Nutritional Support

☐ **8. Evening Primrose Oil (a brand using the "Efamol" form) or borage oil (less expensive):** Take 3000 mg a day for three months and then just the week before your period.

Also aim to eat salmon or tuna at least three times per week. You can also supplement with fish oil. Take 1 to 2 tablets of Vectomega (Europharma) daily.

To Treat Hot Flashes

☐ **9. Black Cohosh (Remifemin by Enzymatic Therapy):** Take two tablets twice a day for two months and then you can lower the dose to one tablet twice a day.

Note: This treatment can take six weeks to work.

SUPPLEMENTS FOR SPECIFIC CONDITIONS COMMON IN SUGAR ADDICTION

Anxiety

☐ **10. Calming Balance (by Health Freedom Nutrition):** Start with three capsules, three times a day. After maximum benefit has been achieved (usually in one to six weeks, though it begins to work within thirty minutes or less), decrease to the minimum dose that provides the same benefit (i.e., two capsules twice a day).

Chronic Fatigue/Fibromyalgia

☐ **11. Energy Revitalization System multivitamin powder (Berry or Citrus by Enzymatic Therapy or Integrative Therapeutics):** Take one-half to one scoop a day (as feels best) blended with milk, water, or yogurt. If diarrhea occurs, mix the powder with milk and/or start with a lower dose and work your way up to the dose that feels best; or, divide the daily dose into smaller doses and take two or three times a day.

☐ **12. Ribose (Bioenergy):** Take one 5-gram scoop of powder three times a day for three weeks, then twice a day. If this is too energizing, take it with milk or food or lower the dose. Effects are usually seen within two to three weeks. Find it at your health food store or at www.endfatigue.com.

☐ **13. Revitalizing Sleep Formula (from Enzymatic Therapies or Integrative Therapeutics):** This formula contains 200 mg of valerian, 90 mg of passionflower, 50 mg of L-theanine, 30 mg of hops, 20 mg of lemon balm, and 28 mg of wild lettuce. Take two to four capsules each night, thirty to sixty minutes before bedtime. It can also be used during the day for anxiety. If valerian energizes you (this occurs in 5 to 10 percent of people), use the other components. It is also excellent for anxiety. Do not take more than eight capsules a day.

☐ **14. Sustained-Release Magnesium (by Jigsaw Health):** If taking magnesium causes diarrhea, use this form (it contains 125 mg per tablet, plus other helpful nutrients).

☐ **14a. Sleep Tonight from Enzymatic Therapy.** The mix of ashwagandha and Phosphatidyl Serine naturally balances adrenal stress hormone levels. Expect to see results after just one week. Take one to two at night.

☐ **15. Adrenal Stress End (from Enzymatic Therapies or Integrative Therapeutics):** This combination product contains important nutrients for adrenal health. Take one or two capsules each morning (or one or two in the morning and another at noon). Lower the dosage or take with food if it upsets your stomach (which is unusual).

For Pain Associated with Chronic Fatigue Syndrome and Fibromyalgia

☐ **15a. End Pain:** This product contains extracts of the herbal remedies boswellia serrata, white willow bark, and cherry fruit. It can be more effective than Celebrex and Motrin and is much safer. Although some effects can be seen immediately, improvement continues to build over a period of six weeks.

☐ **15b. Bos-Curamin from EuroPharma.** This clinically proven blend of BosPure Boswellia BCM-95, a very highly absorbable form of curcumin, (turmeric).

Directions for End Pain and Bos-Curamin: Take one to two tablets of either, or both together, three times a day. It takes two to six weeks to see the full effect, though benefits are often seen in half an hour. These can be taken along with pain medications, allowing the dose of medication to be lowered, or even stopped, over time. Then the dose of the herbal(s) can also be lowered. For those with fibromyalgia, it's more effective to start with two capsules, three times a day for six weeks. Also, add Topical Comfrey (Traumaplant by EuroMedica) to especially painful areas three times a day, as needed.

Depression

☐ **16. Fish Oil Support (Vectomega by Euromedica):** Eat at least 6 ounces (170 g) of salmon or tuna at least four times a week for three to nine months until the depression clears and then as needed. I recommend Vectromega (EuroPharma) in which 1–2 tablets replace 8–16 fish oil capsules. We recommend this brand because many others tend to be rancid and often contain mercury, lead, or other toxins.

☐ **17. Happiness 1-2-3! (by Health Freedom Nutrition):** Take two tablets two or three times a day. Give this herbal mix six weeks to work.

If depression persists despite following the recommended treatments above, or if depression is severe, consult with your doctor about taking prescription antidepressants.

Diabetes

For Diabetic Neuropathy (Nerve Pain)

☐ **18. Lipoic acid:** Take 300 mg twice a day.

☐ **19. Acetyl-l-carnitine:** Take 500 mg two to three times a day. It helps both nerve pain and heart failure.

Heart Disease

☐ **20. Ribose (by Bioenergy):** A powder that looks and tastes like sugar (but is healthy and has a negative, very healthy value on the glycemic index), ribose is a key to energy production in the body, including the heart. Take one scoop (5 grams) three times a day for six weeks, then twice a day thereafter. You can find it at www.endfatigue.com.

☐ **21. Coenzyme Q10:** Coenzyme Q10 is critical for energy production. This nutrient is especially important for anyone on cholesterol-lowering "statin" medications (i.e., Lipitor), even if there is no heart problem, because these medications cause coenzyme Q10 deficiency. Take 400 mg a day for six weeks, then 200 mg a day. Use the 200 mg chewable Smart Q10 wafers from Enzymatic Therapy.

☐ **22. Magnesium Orotate:** Take 6,000 mg a day for one month, then 3,000 mg a day.

☐ **23. Fish Oil support (Vectomega by Euromedia):** Take 1 to 2 tablets a day. We recommend this brands because many others tend to be rancid and often contain mercury, lead, or other toxins. In addition, 1 to 2 tablets of Vectomega replaces 8 to 16 fish oil capsules.

Hypothyroidism

☐ **24. BMR Complex (thyroid glandular plus tyrosine, iodine, and other thyroid-supporting nutrients, available from Integrative Therapeutics):** Take one or two capsules three times daily between meals or as feels best.

☐ **25.** Breast cysts, cancer, or tenderness suggest that iodine deficiency is contributing to your low thyroid condition, and we recommend taking either **Tri-iodine** (Terry Naturally by EuroPharma, which is kelp-based, see www.europharmausa.com) or **Iodoral** (by Optimox, see www.optimox.com). Take one tablet or capsule a day for two to four months. Each tablet or capsule contains 6.25 mg of iodine.

☐ **25a. Iron:** If your ferritin level is under 60, I give 30 to 60 mg of iron a day, making sure that the supplement also has at least 100 mg of vitamin C to enhance absorption. If you can't tolerate iron supplements, Flora Dix makes a liquid iron supplement that has 11 mg of iron per dose (take one to two doses a day), is well absorbed, and does not upset the stomach.

Don't take iron within six hours of thyroid hormone preparations or Cipro (antibiotic), as this prevents their absorption. Take on an empty stomach. It is okay to miss up to three doses a week. Stop in four to six months or when your ferritin blood test is over 60. Iron may turn your stool black.

IBS/Spastic Colon

☐ **26. Peppermint Oil:** Take one or two enteric/stomach-coated 0.2 cc capsules three times a day between meals (not with food) for spastic colon. I recommend Peppermint Plus from Enzymatic Therapies or Mentharil from Integrative Therapeutics.

☐ **27. Simethicone (Mylicon, available over-the-counter in most pharmacies or food markets):** Chew 40 to 80 mg three times a day as needed for abdominal gas pain.

Indigestion

☐ **28. Complete GEST Digestive Enzymes (from Enzymatic Therapies):** Take two capsules with each meal to help you digest your food properly. Also drink warm liquids (not cold drinks) with meals because digestive enzymes (including those made by your body) work only in warm temperatures. If the enzymes irritate your stomach, wait until your stomach feels better before resuming the enzymes. Only use plant-based (not animal-based) digestive enzymes to aid digestion.

☐ **29. DGL Licorice (Advanced DGL):** Take 380 mg (not the sugar-free variety). Chew one capsule twice daily, twenty minutes before meals, over a period of one to two months, and then as needed.

☐ **30. Mastic gum:** Take 500 to 1000 mg twice a day for one to two months to help your stomach heal from indigestion, then if needed for recurrences.

☐ **31. Limonene, plus Sea Buckthorne (Heartburn Free by Enzymatic Therapy or Advanced Heartburn Rescue by Europharma).** Take this to treat an *H. pylori* infection (a common problem aggravating indigestion) and to heal your stomack lining. Once your indigestion is better as a result of taking DGL licorice and/or mastic gum, take one pill of limonene every day for 2 months, then as needed. This may give long-term relief after taking only a single two month course.

Migraines and Tension Headaches

To Prevent and Treat Migraines

☐ **32. Butterbur (Petadolex by Enzymatic Therapy):** Take 50 mg three times a day for one month and then 50 mg twice a day thereafter to prevent migraines. You can take 100 mg every three hours to eliminate an acute migraine.

☐ **33. Sustained-Release Magnesium (by Jigsaw Health):** If taking magnesium causes diarrhea, use this form (it contains 125 mg per tablet, plus other helpful nutrients).

☐ **34. Fish Oil Support (Vectomosa by Europharma):** Take 1 to 2 tablets a day. Or eat 6 ounces (170 g) of salmon or tuna at least four times a week for three to nine months until the migraines resolve and then as needed. We recommend this brand because many others tend to be rancid and often contain mercury, lead, or other toxins. In addition, 1 to 2 Vectomega tablets replace 8–16 fish oil capsules.

☐ **35. Coenzyme Q10:** Coenzyme Q10 is critical for energy production. Take 200 mg a day. Use the 200 mg Smart Q10 chewable wafers from Enzymatic Therapy.

☐ **36. Energy Revitalization System Vitamin Powder:** This supplies riboflavin, magnesium, and other nutrients that can markedly decrease the frequency of migraine headaches. **Note:** Give this product six weeks to work.

To Treat Tension Headaches

☐ **37. End Pain (by Enzymatic Therapy) or Pain Formula (by Integrative Therapeutics) herbal mix:** Take three tablets immediately, up to eight a day for headache. For ongoing pain in general, take two tablets three times a day for six weeks to see the full effect. You can then lower it to the dose needed to control the pain.

Osteoporosis

☐ **38. Bone Health (by Ultraceuticals):** Take three tablets twice a day. When bone density normalizes, you can lower the dose to three tablets a day at bedtime. Do not take within three hours of taking thyroid hormone. Bone Health is available at www.vitality101.com.

☐ **38a. OsteoStrong (EuroPharma).** Take four tablets per day plus two strontium capsules per day (available from www.europharmausa.com).

Sinusitis

☐ **39. Sinusitis Nose Spray (prescription):** This formula contains Diflucan, xylitol, Bactroban, bismuth, and triamcinolone. Squirt one or two sprays into each nostril twice a day for six to twelve weeks. If it irritates your nose, use nasal saline spray just before using the prescription spray. Use with the Silver Nose Spray below. It is available by prescription from ITC Compounding Pharmacy (www.itcpharmacy.com, 303-663-4224. See appendix D).

☐ **40. Silver Nose Spray (Argentyn 23 brand by Natural-Immunogenics):** Squirt five to ten sprays into each nostril three times a day for seven to fourteen days until the sinusitis resolves.

APPENDIX B

GLYCEMIC INDEX INFORMATION

The glycemic index (GI) tells you which foods raise your blood glucose fastest and highest. This is especially important for sugar addicts to keep in mind. Pure glucose gets a GI score of 100—all other foods are measured in relation to glucose. A food with a glycemic index above 85 raises blood sugar rapidly, but a food with a glycemic index below 30 does not raise your blood sugar much at all. As a sugar addict, you'll want to eat foods that score low on the glycemic index as often as possible.

Classification	GI Range	Examples
Low GI	55 or below	Most fruits and vegetables (except potatoes, water melon), grainy breads, pasta, legumes/pulses, milk, and products extremely low in carbohydrates (fish, eggs, meat, some cheeses, nuts, cooking oil), and brown rice
Medium GI	56–69	Whole wheat products, basmati rice, sweet potatoes, table sugar, and most white rice (e.g., jasmine)
High GI	70 and above	Cornflakes, baked potatoes, watermelon, croissants, white bread, extruded breakfast cereals (e.g., Rice Krispies), and straight glucose (100)

FRESH FRUIT	GLYCEMIC INDEX
Cherries	63
Blueberries (fresh or frozen)	53
Grapes	53
Bananas	52
Oranges	42
Peaches	42
Strawberries (fresh or frozen)	40
Pears	38
Apples	38

FRESH VEGETABLES	GLYCEMIC INDEX
Starchy Vegetables	

These tend to be largely sugar and starch with low protein content to balance the starch, so limit your intake of these to 4 ounces (115 g) or less on most days, using those with a lower glycemic index whenever possible.

Parsnips	97
Potato	High 80's
Rutabaga	72
Beets	64
Sweet potato	61
Corn	53
Carrots	47

Beans and Legumes

Although some beans and legumes score high on the glycemic index, they also are high in protein, vitamins, minerals, and fiber, making them a healthy choice for sugar addicts—especially vegetarians. Enjoy up to two or three servings of these a day.

Unless otherwise noted, the following GI scores refer to dried beans or peas that have been boiled. Canned beans tend to have a higher glycemic index value.

Black-eyed peas	33 to 20
Butter beans	28 to 36, average 31
Chickpeas (garbonzo beans)	31 to 36
Chickpeas, canned	42
Kidney beans	13 to 46, average 34
Lentils	18 to 37
Lentils, canned	52
Navy beans (white beans, haricot)	30 to 39
Navy beans, pressure cooked	29 to 59
Peas, dried, split	32
Pinto beans	39
Pinto beans, canned	45
Soybeans	15 to 20
Soybeans, canned	14

Other Vegetables

Most other vegetables, and particularly green leafy ones, usually score zero or near zero on the glycemic index. Try to eat three to five portions a day, but you can have as much as you like. Vinaigrette or oil and vinegar dressings can be used on salads as desired.

DAIRY PRODUCTS

It's okay to eat up to four servings a day.

Milk, regular (full fat)	11 to 40, average 27
Milk, skim	32
Yogurt without added sugar	14 to 23

BREADS

As you can see, bread has a high glycemic index score. Limit your intake to one or two slices a day or less. We recommend whole-grain products because they have not lost most of their vitamins and minerals through refining and processing.

White bread	71
Whole wheat bread	71
Wheat bread made with 50% cracked wheat kernels	58
Wheat bread made with 75% cracked wheat kernels	48

COLD CEREALS

These tend to have a high glycemic index score. Although a breakfast of eggs and meat (skip the potatoes or grits) is preferable, if you don't have time to prepare this, a bowl of cereal for breakfast is okay as long as it does not contain more than 14 grams of sugar per serving (which equals 3½ teaspoons [14 g] of sugar; read the nutrition information on the box). Cheerios, Life cereal, and Shredded Wheat are good choices.

All-Bran	42
Cornflakes	81
Corn Chex	83
Crispix	87
Fruit Loops	69
Golden Grahams	71
Grape-Nuts	71
Life	66
Puffed Wheat	73
Rice Krispies–type cereals	88
Rice Chex	89
Shredded Wheat	75
Special K	69
	Total 76

PASTA

The glycemic index scores for standard wheat pastas depend on thickness (the thicker the pasta, the lower the GI) and the way it is cooked (al dente—somewhat firm—has the lowest GI). The longer you cook it, the softer it is, and the higher the GI. Eat these sparingly (up to four servings a week).

Most wheat pastas	35 to 60

NUTS

These have a low GI score and you can eat as much as you like. Nuts make good snacks.

Cashews	22
Peanuts	14
Almonds	0
Brazil nuts	0
Hazelnuts	0
Macadamia nuts	0
Pecans	0
Walnuts	0

APPENDIX C

FINDING A PRACTITIONER

Physician Organizations

Holistic physicians are much more likely than conventional, allopathic doctors to be familiar with the treatments and principles discussed in this book. The following organizations include more than 3,000 practitioners throughout North America who take a holistic approach to medicine.

TO FIND A HOLISTIC MD OR DO (DOCTOR OF OSTEOPATHY):

American Board of Integrative Holistic Medicine

www.holisticboard.org or www.ABIHM.org

This board certifies physicians as having advanced training in the use of natural therapies. Their website lists more than 1,000 board-certified holistic physicians.

To find a naturopath who has completed a four-year training program equivalent to medical school:

American Association of Naturopathic Physicians

www.naturopathic.org

More and more states are allowing naturopaths who have graduated from one of the seven naturopathic colleges in North America to prescribe and treat like physicians.

IF YOU HAVE CHRONIC FATIGUE SYNDROME OR FIBROMYALGIA (CFS/FMS)

Instead of trying to teach your doctor how to treat CFS/FMS, go to a specialist. Holistic physicians listed with one of the two organizations above are also more likely to be able to help you than the average physician who may be unfamiliar with these illnesses.

You can also find a doctor who specializes in CFS/FMS by visiting www.vitality101.com and clicking on Physician Finder.

I treat CFS and fibromyalgia patients from around the world, either in person or by phone. I'd be happy to help you recover your health and vitality! For more information, see www.vitality101.com, e-mail office@endfatigue.com, and/or call 410-573-5389.

In addition, the free online Energy Analysis Program at www.endfatigue.com will analyze your medical history (and your laboratory test results, if available) to determine what is most important to optimize energy production in your case. The program will also create a treatment protocol tailored to your case. This will allow you to begin the natural parts of the protocol on your own and will assist and support your doctor in giving you the best possible care.

APPENDIX D

RESOURCES

Also see appendix A for a list of commonly recommended products (usually mixes of natural products), where we've organized them according to addiction type and specific medical conditions to simplify the treatment of sugar addiction and its related problems. Most of these products are available from my website at www.vitality101.com, 800-333-5287, or from health food stores.

This appendix offers many helpful resources, including how to find medications (at the best price) and supplements (retail and wholesale), water filters, excellent compounding pharmacies, and much more.

Allergy Elimination
NAET

714-523-8900

www.NAET.com

This website supplies information about the Nambudripad's Allergy Elimination Technique (NAET), including help with locating practitioners worldwide.

Compounding Pharmacies
ITC Compounding Pharmacy

303-663-4224 or 866-374-0696

www.itcpharmacy.com

This mail-order compounding pharmacy does a superb job of quality control and makes a wide range of bio-identical hormones, topical pain formulas, Sinusitis Nose Spray, and much more.

Prescription Medications
Costco Pharmacy

www.costco.com

Costco also has excellent prices for generic prescriptions. To see what a medication should cost, go to the website above. You do not have to be a Costco member to fill prescriptions at their pharmacy.

Stool Parasite Testing

Genova Diagnostics (previously Great Smokies Diagnostic Laboratory)

800-522-4762

www.gdx.net

This lab does an excellent job with stool testing for ova and parasites (O&P testing) and bacterial infections, as well as many other tests. Genova Diagnostics has performed Optimized Parasite Recovery with experienced microbiology technicians for more than twenty years. Eradication of parasites and treating bacterial overgrowth can be very helpful in addressing the fatigue and bowel symptoms often seen in sugar addicts. Stool-testing kits are available through your doctor, who can order the testing from Genova Diagnostics. Samples are collected at home and sent to Genova Diagnostics. These tests are covered by most insurance policies.

Saunas

High Tech Health International, Inc

800-794-5355

www.hightechhealth.com

Sweating can remove toxins—especially if you shower immediately after taking a sauna—and can be very helpful for maintaining good health. Many of the newer saunas are called "far infrared"—a half-hour session three to seven times a week can aid detoxification. I use and recommend the ones from High Tech Health.

Sinusitis Treatment

888-434-0033 or 303-771-0033

www.sinussurvival.com

www.fullyalivemedicine.com

Dr. Ivker's sinus survival website offers nasal steamers to help heal chronic sinusitis, as well as many other helpful tools and resources. If you are in the Boulder, Co area, Dr. Ivker is now seeing patients again.

Water Filters

Multipure Drinking Water Systems

443-949-0409

www.jacobsonhealth.com

Contact: Bren Jacobson

Consultant for health and environmental concerns, especially water, and distributor of Multi-Pure water filters, Bren Jacobson also does personal counseling for people who are looking for the best mix of natural and standard treatments for their medical problems (available in person or by phone).

Information and Supplements

Jacob Teitelbaum, MD

800-333-5287 or 410-573-5389

www.endfatigue.com

Many of the products recommended in this book, particularly the hard-to-find ones, are available through our website. At our website, you can sign up for free email newsletters that will keep you on the cutting edge of developments in health care—especially issues related to sugar addiction, pain, and fatigue. You'll also find a free online Energy Analysis program for people with chronic fatigue or fibromyalgia that will analyze your symptoms (and your lab results, if available) to tailor a treatment protocol to optimize energy production in your case.

Enzymatic Therapy, Inc

800-783-2286

www.enzy.com

This company produces many excellent products, including the Fatigued to Fantastic! product line, which I developed. This line includes Fatigued to Fantastic! Energy Revitalization System vitamin powder and B complex; Fatigued to Fantastic! Daily Energy B Complex; End Pain; Adrenal Stress End; and Revitalizing Sleep Formula. Enzymatic Therapy products can be found in most health food stores, as well as at www.endfatigue.com.

EuroPharma

866-598-5487

www.europharmausa.com

This company was founded by Terry Lemerond, who's been at the head of innovation in the natural products industry for decades. Their products include Curamin, which is likely the most powerful natural pain remedy in history! Using new natural technologies, they have developed ways to dramatically increase the absorption of nutrients, so that you don't have to take handfuls of pills every day. To find the cutting-edge of natural health, just look for Terry!

Wholesale Products for Health Care Practitioners

Most of the products recommended in this book can be found at www.vitality101.com or most health food stores. Health practitioners or health food stores that would like to carry these products wholesale for the public can contact:

Enzymatic Therapy, Inc.

800-783-2286

www.enzymatictherapy.com

This company sells to health food stores and makes many excellent products, including the Fatigued to Fantastic product line, which I developed. This line includes Fatigued to Fantastic Energy Revitalization System vitamin powder and B-complex, Fatigued to Fantastic Daily Energy B-Complex, and End Pain and Revitalizing Sleep Formula.

The products I've recommended in this book can be found in most health food stores as well as at www.vitality101.com.

Integrative Therapeutics, Inc. (ITI)

800-931-1709

Representative: Cathy Leet

920-737-8828

www.integrativeinc.com

Along with EuroMedia, I feel this is one of the two best companies in the United States making products for health practitioners only, and I am so impressed with them that I asked them to make my End Fatigue line of products. This line includes the Energy Revitalization System vitamin powder (which can replace more than thirty-five different vitamin tablets a day), Daily Energy B-Complex, Pain Formula Herbal Mix, Adrenal Stress End, and Revitalizing Sleep Formula. ITI voluntarily registered with the FDA, so their products have to go through the same testing for potency and purity as pharmaceuticals do. They have many excellent products, and Cathy Leet is great to work with.

Other Products

Body Ecology

800-4-STEVIA or 800-478-3842

www.bodyecology.com

They have the best-tasting stevia I have found. They also offer stevia cookbooks.

Health Freedom Nutrition

800-980-8780

www.hfn-usa.com

Go to this mail-order company for herbals for anxiety or depression. They also make Calming Balance and Happiness 1-2-3! (also available at www.vitality101.com) and have an informative newsletter.

Emerson Ecologice

ITI and Euromdica's complete line of products can also be purchased through their distributor partners:

Emerson Ecologics (EE)
800-654-4432 (Manchester, NH)
800-824-2434 (Redlands, CA)
www.emersonecologics.com
Natural Partners, Inc. (NP)
888-633-7620
www.naturalpartners.com

Natural Partners carries an extensive line of wholesale natural products for health practitioners' offices.

ACKNOWLEDGMENTS

Jacob Teitelbaum: So many special people helped make this book possible that I cannot possibly list them all. In truth, I have created nothing new; I have simply synthesized the wonderful work done by an army of hardworking and courageous physicians and healers.

I would like to extend my sincerest thanks to:

First and foremost Laurie, my wife, for her patience with me during the writing of this book. My mom and dad, who continue to inspire me despite having passed on long ago. To my co-author Chrystle Fiedler, who took my knowledge and crafted it into a book that everyone can use to beat their own sugar addiction.

To my staff, especially Cheryl Alberto, who keep everything handled while I'm busy writing and teaching. Their hard work, compassion, and dedication (and, I must admit, patience with me) are what make my work possible.

My wonderful, amazing, and dedicated publicist and friend, Dean Draznin, and his staff, including Terri Slater and Dawn Saffrit, who are my teammates in making effective treatment and health available to everyone. A special thanks also to Richard Crouse and Rich Mendelson, my computer "genies." Whenever I just wish for stuff, they make it happen!

The Anne Arundel Medical Center librarian, Joyce Miller. Over the last 30 years, I have often wondered when she would politely tell me to stop asking for so many studies. So far, she has not. In fact, she always smiles when I ask her for more.

Bren Jacobson and Dr. Alan Weiss who keep me intellectually, emotionally, and spiritually honest while reminding me to reclaim my sense of humor.

Chrystle Fiedler: I'm grateful to have taken this journey with Jacob Teitelbaum, MD, (Dr. T!) a one of a kind, doctor, healer and teacher. Many thanks go to Marilyn Allen of the Allen O'Shea Literary Agency for her support and guidance. Special thanks go to the editorial team at Fair Winds Press, especially senior editor Jill Alexander.

ABOUT THE AUTHORS

Jacob Teitelbaum, M.D., is an Internal Medicine specialist who has treated sugar-related issues, including chronic fatigue and pain, for over 30 years. He is Medical Director of the International Practioners Alliance Network (www.vitality101.com/PAN) and author of the free iPhone application "Cures A-Z." Teitelbaum is senior author of the landmark studies "Effective Treatment of Chronic Fatigue Syndrome and Fibromyalgia—a Placebo-controlled Study" and "Effective Treatment of CFS & Fibromyalgia with D-Ribose," and author of the best-selling book *From Fatigued to Fantastic!* (3rd revised edition, Avery/Penguin Group) and *Pain Free 1-2-3—A Proven Program for Eliminating Chronic Pain Now* (McGraw-Hill). He does frequent media appearances including *Good Morning America*, CNN, Fox News Channel, *The Dr. Oz Show*, and *Oprah & Friends* with Dr. Mehmet Oz. He lives in Kona, Hawaii. His websites are www.vitality101.com and www.endfatigue.com.

Deirdre Rawlings, Ph.D., N.D., M.H., C.N.C., is a healthy-cooking coach and the founder of Nutri-Living, a holistic nutrition practice focusing on psycho-nutritional counseling. She is the author of *Foods That Help with the Battle Against Fibromyalgia*.

Chrystle Fiedler has written over a hundred articles on health topics for many national publications including *Natural Health*, *Sprituality & Health*, *Woman's Day*, *Better Homes & Gardens*, *Prevention*, *Arthritis Today*, *Remedy*, *Vegetarian Times*, and *Health* magazine. Chrystle is the author of *The Complete Idiot's Guide to Natural Remedies* (Alpha 2009) and the co-author of *The Country Almanac of Home Remedies* (Fair Winds Press, 2011) and *The Home Reference to Holistic Health and Healing* (2015) with herbalist Brigitte Mars. Chrystle also writes a natural remedies mystery series for Gallery Books/Simon & Schuster, including the books, *Death Drops*, *Scent to Kill* and *The Garden of Death* (March 2015). Learn more about her at: www.chrystlefiedler.com.

INDEX

thyroid stimulating test
(TSH) and, 178

hypothyroidism
action plan summary, 184
adrenal glands and, 25
calcium and, 215
cravings and, 63
depression and, 153
diagnosing, 177, 178
Hashimoto's thyroiditis
and, 178
heart function and,
180, 183
iodine and, 182–183
irritable bowel syndrome
(IBS) and, 186
long-term effects of, 177
menopause and, 125
miscarriage and, 179
natural therapies, 182–183
nutrition and, 182
prescription medications,
180–182
small intestinal bacterial
overgrowth (SIBO)
and, 189
symptoms of, 177
testosterone
supplementation
and, 130
thyroid hormone and, 179
treatment risks, 183
weight and, 207, 210

I

immune system. See also
infections.
antibodies and, 8
chronic fatigue syndrome
(CFS), 139, 146
cortisol and, 24, 25
fibromyalgia (FMS) and, 146
function of, 8
inflammation and, 8
nutrition and, 18

sleep and, 30
support, 101–102
yeast overgrowth and, 29,
30, 31

indigestion
action plan summary, 195
antacids and, 192, 195
digestive enzymes,
192–194
licorice, 194
mastic gum, 194–195
stomach acid and, 192
stomach infections
and, 195
treatment of, 194

infections. See also immune
system.
chronic fatigue syndrome
(CFS) and, 146
fibromyalgia (FMS) and, 146
hand-washing and, 65
hydration and, 64
irritable bowel syndrome
(IBS) and, 188
sleep and, 64
stomach infections
and, 195
support, 63–64

inflammation
food allergies and, 30
immune system and, 8
support, 150, 166

insomnia. See also sleep.
Ambien and, 62
Bach Flower Remedies, 58
caffeine and, 17
cortisol and, 24
Flexeril and, 62
lavender and, 59, 60
lemon balm and, 58
Neurontin and, 62
passionflower and, 59
prescription medications, 62
progesterone and, 37

Revitalizing Sleep Formula, 59
theanine and, 58
trazodone and, 62
valerian and, 59
wild lettuce and, 58

insulin
adrenal glands and, 23, 24
chromium and, 50, 83
function of, 35, 161
glutathione, 85
testosterone and, 128

insulin resistance. See also
diabetes.
andropause and, 39
diabetes and, 35, 161
diagnosing, 211
exercise and, 163
long-term effects of, 160
magnesium and, 72
menopause and, 36
omega-3 fatty acids and, 51
serotonin and, 39
sleep and, 56
testosterone and, 36, 211
vitamin D and, 73
weight and, 36, 161, 163,
167, 206, 210–211

irritable bowel syndrome (IBS)
antacids and, 189–190
elimination diets and, 187
food sensitivity and, 187
fructose and, 187
hypothalamus and,
185–186
hypothyroidism and, 186
infections and, 188
lactose and, 187
natural remedies, 189–190
peppermint oil and, 188
small intestinal bacterial
overgrowth (SIBO)
and, 189
summary action plan, 190
yeast overgrowth and, 186